WITHDRAWN

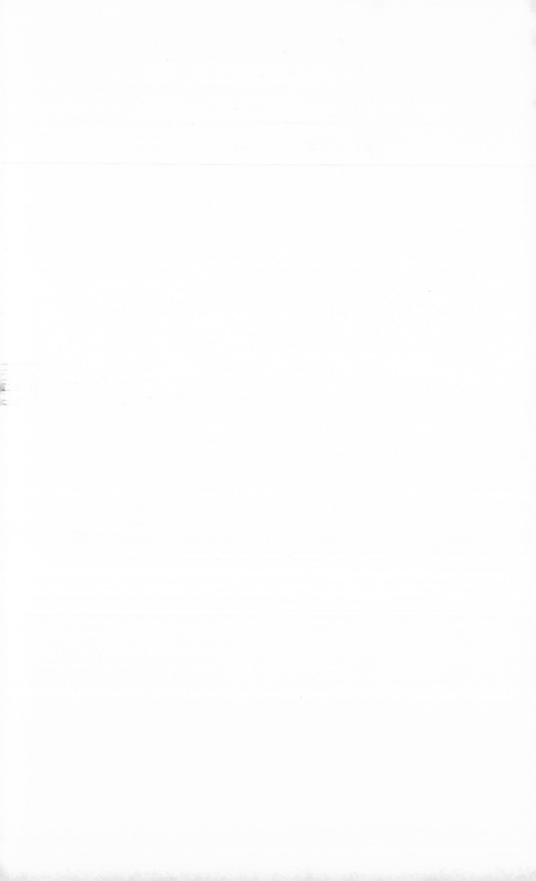

RESTORYING
OUR
LIVES

RESTORYING
OUR
LIVES

Personal Growth Through Autobiographical Reflection

Gary M. Kenyon and William L. Randall

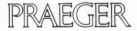

Westport, Connecticut
London

Library of Congress Cataloging-in-Publication Data

Kenyon, Gary M.
    Restorying our lives / personal growth through autobiographical
reflection / Gary M. Kenyon and William L. Randall.
        p.   cm.
    Includes bibliographical references and index.
    ISBN 0–275–95663–6 (alk. paper)
    1. Autobiography.   2.   Autobiography—Psychological aspects.
I. Randall, William Lowell, 1950–   . II. Title.
CT25.K36   1997
808′.06666692—dc21   97–5587

British Library Cataloguing in Publication Data is available.

Copyright © 1997 by Gary M. Kenyon and William L. Randall

All rights reserved. No portion of this book may be
reproduced, by any process or technique, without the
express written consent of the publisher.

Library of Congress Catalog Card Number: 97–5587
ISBN: 0–275–95663–6

First published in 1997

Praeger Publishers, 88 Post Road West, Westport, CT 06881
An imprint of Greenwood Publishing Group, Inc.

Printed in the United States of America

The paper used in this book complies with the
Permanent Paper Standard issued by the National
Information Standards Organization (Z39.48–1984).

10 9 8 7 6 5 4 3 2 1

Contents

Preface

"That's the *story* of my life!" we sometimes sigh. Often a sign of frustration with patterns that dog our affairs, it can also betray bemused affection for the peculiar course our life seems to take overall. In this book, we play with the implications of the familiar but fascinating metaphor behind such an expression: life as story. In effect, we use this metaphor as a lens to examine some of the unsung aspects of continuity and change in both our lives and our relationships. In this preface, though, we want to say something about the story of the book itself.

First, writing it has been a *dialogical* process, where "dialogue" means a conversation across differences. Each of us has brought to it particular questions and a particular lifestory. Though our stories—plus the thrusts of our respective previous writings—intersect in significant ways (making us compatible colleagues), they are none the less distinct. The "gospels" according to Kenyon and Randall are not identical. We do not agree on every point, nor have we tried to write with a seamless style or single voice. Far from seeing such differences as weaknesses, however, we view them as strengths. In a sense, you are getting three books in one. Besides the two books each of us thought to write on our own (and they will hover in the wings) is the one work that resulted from the countless conversations and delicate debates that we enjoyed—and required—to synthesize our visions.

If writing this book has been a dialogical process, no less should be reading it. "Dialogical" in the sense that we raise more issues than we resolve, issues you may find yourself pondering for some time to come. Thus, we have sprinkled the book with numerous practical questions which, considered on your own or with others, can help you relate our key concepts to your own experience. These questions, adapted from workshops and courses we have developed over the years, give the book the flavor of a *work*book in some respects. Ultimately, though, it is a book less about technique than about perspective, a perspective that appreciates certain overlooked intricacies of the "inside" of being human and contributes needed insights to more technical approaches concerned with "solving" particular "problems," whether in therapy, health care, or education.

Second, writing this book has been an *interdisciplinary* process. This is because a story is by nature an interdisciplinary entity. It is "about" many things at once—relationships (psychology and sociology), values and beliefs (ethics and philosophy), making a living (economics and accounting), eating and drinking (chemistry and biology), learning and loving and making sense of the world (education and spirituality). For both these reasons, writing *about* story necessarily crosses disciplined lines. In short, our method is consistent with our metaphor.

But life, too, is never about any one subject. Thus, traditional academic programs can be rather frustrating, for in order to render life comprehensible, they are forever dividing it into so many conquerable "fields." By bringing life into interface with story—as we do when we entertain the book's central concept *lifestory* (two words we treat as one, like *history*)— we are thus being doubly interdisciplinary. But, intellectually, this is hardly a problem. Indeed, most helping professionals are continually confronted by the un-discipline-d dimensions of their work. Such dimensions the story metaphor can accommodate with comparative ease, thus enabling us to honor the individuals with whom we deal not as "cases" or sets of "deficits" but as persons who are in their own way already whole and merely trying to find their path through the maze of the world.

Third, writing this book has been an *experimental* process, not just because it is a collaborative venture (inspired by the belief that two heads are at least as good as one) but also because we are testing a hypothesis. Our hypothesis is that giving someone the space and encouragement to lay out their lifestory, then to stand back and assess both its content and its form *as a story*, affords them an affectionate distance on the shape of their life as they have composed it hitherto, with its many "chapters," "characters," and "themes," and the several twists and turns in its "plot." It thus affords them a peculiarly liberating self-acceptance. *This is my story*, it enables them to claim; *such as it is, it has an integrity all its own.* Such distance and acceptance are essential to self-care. They are certainly necessary to autobiographical reflection, and thus to personal growth. Hence our subtitle.

In constructing this hypothesis, we have in mind primarily those whose role is to *facilitate* such growth, whether as professionals or not: anyone (clinician or counselor, pastor or teacher, relative or friend) who works with people directly, accompanies them on the path to personal change, and invites them to greater insight into themselves and their relationships. If you will, we want to "help people help people help themselves" by laying out with the least jargon possible a process of storytelling and storylistening through which we can act as coauthors of each other's lives. While we do not purport to thereby answer all of humanity's ills, we hope we offer a valuable tool for carrying out this intricate yet honorable role.

As to our right to write on such a subject, one of us—Gary—is a philosopher-gerontologist who has focused on "metaphors of aging" (Kenyon et al., 1991) and, more recently, on "biographical aging" (Birren et al., 1996). The other—Bill—is an adult educator, former parish minister, and one-time English instructor who has become fascinated by "the stories we *are*" (Randall, 1995). Together, our principal "expertise" lies in playing with "the narrative root metaphor" (Sarbin, 1986b) and thinking about everyday life as a storied affair, and inviting others to do the same. In doing so, we are repeatedly struck by the appeal such thinking possesses—the current epidemic of "storytelling circles" and "storyfests" being a case in point. It is our belief that understanding the poetic, aesthetic, and even spiritual complexity of our own lives is vital to helping others fathom the complexity of theirs. For this reason, again, we have laced the book with questions that invite not just professionals but indeed *any* of us to take stock of our stories and the roles they play in the lives we lead.

Dialogical, interdisciplinary, experimental—all three come to mind as we think of the people who have helped us transform this book from dream to reality. For Gary, that includes Liz, Jessica, and Christina and the students of "Aging and Biography." It also includes Jim Birren, Michael Chandler, and Kjell Rubenson, three mentors who, through their sustained encouragement and support, have made it possible for him to wander on his chosen trail. For Bill, it includes his sister Carol, Paula Caplan, and David Flynn for their encouragement, and the students of a course that, each time it is offered, seems to acquire a different name, be it "Life Story and Self-Creation" or "Narrative Gerontology." For Gary and Bill both, it includes Gary and Bill both, as well as Penny Granter, our departmental secretary; Jan-Erik Ruth, friend and fellow narrativist, who made numerous helpful suggestions; Cheryl Cormier and Kathy Geldart, who offered feedback on earlier drafts; and our common home, St. Thomas University. Without the continual testing of ideas we enjoy with colleagues both there and beyond, we might have failed to get this story out. Before we proceed, though, we want to outline what follows.

Storytelling is as old as language itself. Therefore, to write about restorying our lives is not just to go along with the academic "flavor of the month." Yet, in a sense, it is. In the literature review we provide in Chapter 1, for instance, we show how much material has been written on this subject during the last two decades. Also in Chapter 1, and in Chapter 2 as well, we examine the underlying characteristics and theoretical assumptions that form the life as story metaphor. This includes a discussion of what it means to look at our lives as stories, and the implications and limitations of this view. Then, in Chapter 3, we focus on the characteristics of the metaphor itself, exploring the myriad of stories within and around us. Chapter 4 proceeds to look closely at the process of "composing a life" and the role played in it by the actual components of stories, such as plot, character, point of view, genre, and setting. In Chapter 5, we examine the process of *re*storying our lives and the principal resources for carrying it out: education, spirituality, therapy, art, other people, and our own selves.

Following this look at ourselves as both stories and agents of restorying, we consider in Chapter 6 a number of important ethical issues concerning the use of the story metaphor, drawing examples from the field of gerontology where the lifestory approach has special relevance. In particular, we reflect on the issue of proper and improper settings for biographical encounters. In some settings, for example, storylistening may be an ethical obligation, while in others it may be inappropriate. Finally, in Chapter 7 we ponder the implications, and speculate on future directions, of understanding our lives in storied terms, guided by the conviction that, in a postmodern world, our lifestories are central to the discovery and creation of personal meaning.

Organized in such a manner, then, this book explores the rich contribution of "the story of my life" to a number of dimensions at once, from the personal to the professional and from the practical to the philosophical.

Chapter 1

Introduction

We are the stories we like to tell.

Roger Schank (1990)

THE CONCEPT

In this book, we present a fresh way of understanding what it means to be a person. To be a person is to have a story. More than that, it is to *be* a story. For those of you who "work with" persons, we thus present a fresh way of understanding what that work involves. Whether you are a social worker, counselor, or educator, a health care professional or caring friend, we offer you (literally) a *novel* image for helping other people. We call it "restorying" lives.

Restorying is a complex process, indeed an aesthetic process, for it concerns the shape we assign to our experience overall. In a sense, it is a poetic process, where "poetic" derives from *poeisis*, a Greek word for "making by imagination into words" (Hillman, 1975, p. 124). From poeisis, we also get "poetics," which means the study of the literary arts—or literary theory. Restorying, we could say, is the *literary* process of re-composing the stories we have "made up" about who we are, where we have come from, and where we are headed.

But restorying is a process in which you can play a powerful role: as *agents* of restorying, "biographical coaches" (Alheit, 1995), coauthors of the stories by which other people live. Your skills in listening and caring can assist them profoundly as they weave lifestories that are healthier and more livable. Not only that, but in so assisting them you will likely be restoried yourselves. By a kind of psychological "uncertainty principle," the very act of intervening in their lives changes both them and you.

While this book is about helping others, then, it is also about helping ourselves. In a sense, it is about *healing* ourselves. To invoke a cliché in the world of self-help, it is about being our own best therapists. Undergirding it is the belief that we do not always need to look to experts for whatever wisdom and meaning we may seek in our lives—a belief that runs counter to dominant thinking in modern culture. Nor need we lean, unthinkingly, on the many "master narratives" that until *post*modern times have been our primary resources for making sense of our lives: those overriding, ready-made stories about the world as a whole such as are offered by the world's great faiths.

Our point is not that religion per se is unimportant; only that if it is to be an authentic part of our lives, we must not bow blindly to its authority. Rather, we must assume authorship for how its vision gets woven into our own. Ultimately, the richest resource for meaning and healing is one we already possess. It rests (mostly untapped) in the material of our own lifestory, in the sprawling, many-layered "text" that has been accumulating within us across the years, weaving itself in the depths of, and *as,* our life. If we have eyes to see, plus the courage to inquire within, we can appreciate this text as sacred (Charmé, 1984), as the most meaning-filled "novel" there is—for us. We can learn to "read" it as, so to speak, the greatest story ever told, unfolding right under our nose. Just as we can learn from our encounters with great literature, so can we learn life-changing lessons by turning to the texts of our own experience.

In all these respects, the perspective we propose is a *therapoetic* one. It is a therapy not so much for dealing with psychopathology—that is not our expertise—as for savoring the aesthetic richness of everyday life. If you will, it is a therapy for the sane. In it, storytelling (and storylistening) is not merely a method for solving particular problems that crop up in our lives, but has an importance and integrity all its own, as a means to personal wholeness. In this sense, it is a spiritual activity. Through it, we become more of who we are—"more authentic and more alive" (Atkinson, 1995, p. 51)—and discover and celebrate our personal, ordinary wisdom.

In sum, the thesis of this book is that what we call our life is essentially a set of stories we tell ourselves about our past, present, and future. However, these stories are far from fixed, direct accounts of what happens in our lives, but products of the inveterate fictionalizing of our memory and imagination. That is, we "story" our lives. Moreover, we *re*-story them too. In fact, restorying goes on continually within us. From time to time, it goes on intentionally as well, even radically. Understanding—and stimulating—such restorying is the focus of this book.

THE CONTEXT

We would be immediately remiss if we gave the impression that the notion of restorying has come out of nowhere, or that we thought it up on our own. Quite the opposite is the case, and so we wish here to sketch the context of our work by acknowledging some of the many voices in the many fields that are heralding the compelling conceptual power of "the *story* of my life."

First, the field of psychology. In 1986, in *Actual Minds, Possible Worlds*, Jerome Bruner proposed that philosophers, educators, and psychologists have traditionally focussed on only one mode of thinking of which humans are capable—logical or paradigmatic thought. They have thus ignored another, more basic mode: narrative thought. In his musings on the need for a "psychology of literature" (p. 4), Bruner set forth the features of each. The former, which lies at the heart of the scientific method, "leads to good theory, tight analysis, logical proof, sound argument, and empirical discovery guided by reasoned hypothesis." The latter, which "deals with the vicissitudes of human intention" and lies at the heart of everyday life, "leads instead to good stories, gripping drama, believable (though not necessarily 'true') historical accounts" (pp. 13, 17). In 1987, Bruner built on this distinction in an article on "Life as Narrative" in which he stressed that "a life as lived is inseparable from a life as told" (p. 31); that "we *become* the autobiographical narratives by which we 'tell about' our lives" (p. 15). In a 1990 book, *Acts of Meaning*, he critiqued the growing field of cognitive science (ironically, a field he helped found) for overlooking such insights by ignoring the narrative mode and by succumbing instead to the model of mind as computer.

The same year as *Acts of Meaning*, cognitive scientist Roger Schank (1990) published *Tell Me a Story*, in which (again ironically) he argued that if we want computers to think like humans, we must program them not to process information but to tell stories. Indeed, "story" is central to the three terms around which his argument turns: knowledge, intelligence, and memory. "Knowledge," he says, "is experiences and stories, and intelligence is the apt use of experience and the creation and telling of stories. Memory is memory for stories, and the major processes of memory are the creation, storage, and retrieval of stories" (p. 16).

A further irony, as an aside, is that in 1983 B. F. Skinner published Part 3 of his autobiography. Skinner is considered the father of Behaviorism, a school of thinking that has dominated much of modern psychology and assumes that human beings are essentially reactive victims of environmental and other forms of conditioning. Any attempt to peer into the "black box" of the human mind and attribute importance to such supposed internal states as thoughts and feelings is pointless—a view that thus makes it rather self-contradictory to refer to these states in the course of composing (and musing on) the story of one's life!

In 1986, Theodore Sarbin edited *Narrative Psychology: The Storied Nature of Human Conduct*, a collection of articles that take the narrative root metaphor as their common starting point. Two years later saw the publication of Donald Polkinghorne's *Narrative Knowing and the Human Sciences* (1988), which surveys the origins and influences of this metaphor in relation to a broad range of theories and practices in both the social sciences and the humanities, including history and literature. As the title indicates, his guiding vision reflects that of Bruner, centering on narrative knowing as the fundamental way in which we make sense of our lives in time, of the relationships between events, and of the links between intentions and actions, causes and effects. (See Polkinghorne, 1996.)

Given the growing openness to the storied nature of our lives, or to what the philosopher Santayana once called *literary psychology* (Kerby, 1991), it is not surprising that the narrative perspective spread from academic psychology to psychotherapy and psychoanalysis. Indeed, numerous practitioners had sensed for some time the essence of their work as a controlled process of storytelling, storylistening, and, as it were, story-fixing. Says Frederick Wyatt, "[we] psychoanalysts have known all along that we are dealing in stories and with stories all the time; that we offer ourselves to listen to stories and thereby call them forth; and that through a method contrived for this purpose we can carry listening to a point where it transforms storytelling into the life history of a person" (1986, p. 193). Noteworthy here is the work of Freudian psychoanalyst Roy Schafer, on "narration in the psychoanalytic dialogue" (1980), on analysis as a form of literary criticism (1989), and on "retelling a life" (1992). For Schafer, "each analysis amounts in the end to retelling a life in the past and present—and as it may be in the future. A life," he says, "is re-authored as it is co-authored" (1992, p. xv).

In 1982, another Freudian, Donald Spence, published a pivotal work critiquing the complex process of the telling-listening exchange at the heart of psychoanalysis. In it, he argues that, in this process, narrative truth is a far more relevant (and accessible) goal than historical truth. Rather than *re*constructing a patient's past in the manner of an *archeologist* of the psyche (the guiding metaphor for Freud's own work), Spence insists that psychoanalysis is a process of *con*struction instead. Accordingly, the analyst's task is "to turn the patient's life into a meaningful story" (p. 123); to transform "symptoms, fantasies, and other seemingly random aspects of the patient's behavior into a story with a central theme, a recognizable structure, and an overall sense of coherence" (p. 232). Echoing these insights from a different theoretical perspective is Jungian analyst James Hillman. Writing about what he calls "the fictional side of human nature" (1975, p. 128), Hillman stresses that analysis itself is always a "battle of stories" (p. 139)—the analyst's against the analysand's.

In *Every Person's Life Is Worth a Novel*, Erving Polster (1987) puts a more positive spin on the therapist-client interaction. For Polster, the therapist's function is like the novelist's "in making a big deal out of small selections from all that is happening, taking each event not only for its own sake but also for its meaning in an enlarged perspective" (p. 14). In *The Hero Within*, another therapist, Carol Pearson (1989), stresses that "we make stories about the world and to a large degree live out their plots" (p. xx). In *The Story of Your Life*, therapist Mandy Aftel (1996) takes the story metaphor even more at face value, inviting her readers to take its "entailments" (Lakoff and Johnson, 1980), specifically plot and character, narrator and author, and apply them to understanding our lives. As we do, we can begin (in the words of her subtitle) *becoming the author of our experience*. Social workers Michael White and David Epston (1990), who also identify with the story model, have sparked a conceptual revolution in the field of family therapy with their view of the therapeutic process *per se* as fundamentally a "restorying of experience."

Fascination with the story metaphor is growing among gerontologists examining the biographical (as distinct from biological) aspects of the aging process. Their focus is on the inside of aging—on how, as we advance in years, our lifestory changes in our imagination and creates a shift in our involvement in reminiscence, life review, and other forms of autobiographical reflection. Indeed, in a work entitled *Aging and Biography* (Birren et al., 1996), "story" plays a central role in the articles included. Among these is a review of the use of stories and other biographical materials in psychology and sociology (Ruth and Kenyon, 1996), as well as in several areas of practice, including nursing and community care. One of the editors of the volume is James Birren, who with Donna Deutchman has written on the use of "guided autobiography" with elderly people, a process we discuss in later chapters which invites them to trace certain themes throughout their life (Birren and Deutchman, 1991). Sharon Kaufman (1986) takes such a thematic approach in her study of *The Ageless Self*. Finally, in the work of Kotre (1990), McAdams (1988, 1994, 1996), Atkinson (1995), and Randall (1995, 1996), lifestory is the guiding concept in their respective reflections on life-span development.

From a different source, Joseph Campbell has invited a whole generation of anthropologists and other scholars to celebrate *The Power of Myth* (Campbell and Moyers, 1988). Stephen Larsen (1990), Feinstein, Krippner, and Granger (1988), and Sam Keen (1988, 1993), for example, have all taken their cue from Campbell in stressing the importance of fashioning our own personal mythology. But more mainstream anthropologists have also been affected by the story model. Victor Turner and Edward Bruner, for instance, have critiqued the storying tendencies at work in their discipline, describing it as essentially "a genre of storytelling" (E. Bruner, 1986, p. 139). In other words, "ethnographies are guided by an implicit narrative structure, by a story we tell about the peoples we study" (p. 139).

Among philosophers of history, debate has naturally abounded about the relationships between event and interpretation, reality and story. Though their journey into such relationships is not for us to follow here, some of the thinkers participating in the theoretical fray include Hayden White (1980), Paul Ricouer (1980), and David Carr (1986). A comment by Arthur Danto (1985) typifies the hermeneutical issue raised by the "emplotment" in which historians are inevitably involved. "Historians have motives for making historical statements about one past thing rather than another," he says. "Such attitudes induce [them] to make emphases, to overlook certain things, indeed to distort" (p. 31).

In religious studies, scholars have also wrestled with the story-reality issue. Their ponderings date back to at least 1971, a year that marked the publication of an article by Stephen Crites on "The Narrative Quality of Experience," and of Michael Novak's insightful analysis of autobiography and faith in *Ascent of the Mountain, Flight of the Dove*. Since then, works by scholars such as James Wiggins (1975), Sally TeSelle (1975), Stanley Hauerwas (1977), George Stroup (1981), Hauerwas and Jones (1989), and Don Cupitt (1991) have kept alive a discussion that in many ways was launched by Yale theologian H. Richard Niebuhr.

In *The Meaning of Revelation*, Niebuhr (1941) grapples with the complex relationship—for Judeo-Christians at least—between "faith history" and history per se, or between the inside and outside of the history such believers claim is central to their view of the world, its creation and redemption.

Following Niebuhr, a parade of scholars have grappled with the implications, belief-wise, of the fact that at the core of what Jews and Christians
consider sacred scripture lies not a set of timeless truths but a loose linkage
of myths and legends, chronicles and prophecies, half-histories and pseudo-
biographies concerning a variety of groups and individuals whose experiences are taken as testimony to divine activity in the world.

In education, interest in the story metaphor has been swelled by many
currents. From language arts has come an appreciation of the power of
stories to move the moral imagination and influence the formation of
character in the student exposed to their wisdom (see Rosen, 1986; Coles,
1989; Gold, 1990). From the field of teacher preparation has come a passion
to understand the developing themes in the "narratives of experience" of
student interns as they articulate the process of growing into their role
(Connelly and Clandinin, 1988). From adult education has come a respect
for "the stories lives tell" (Witherell and Noddings, 1991), for "biographical
learning" (Alheit, 1995), and for the narrative complexity of past experience, both our principal resource in, and resistance to, the learning process
(Randall, 1995). Respect has also come for the degree to which transformative learning is inseparable from reworking the myth with which we
understand our place in the world (see Daloz, 1986).

The study of story has been especially intense in the field of literary
theory. There, influenced by insights into the complex exchange between
author, text, and reader (Rosenau, 1992), the simple question "what *is* a
story?" has emerged as both the easiest to state and hardest to resolve
(Leitch, 1986). In turn, it has yielded still thornier questions regarding the
nature of language, the relation between language and learning, and those
aspects of our imagination to which the conventions of stories—plot,
character, and so forth—have a stubborn appeal. We shall say more on this
in a moment as we look at the peculiar challenge, yet openness, to story that
comes under the banner of "postmodernism."

One source of the narrative turn is gender studies. Implicit, and often
explicit, in the literature of this field is a sensitivity to the narrative structure
of personal identity and the pivotal role of storytelling in everyday life. From
her study of storytelling within families, for instance, sociologist Elizabeth
Stone (1988) argues that "family stories—telling them and listening to
them—belong more to the women's sphere. . . . the family is essentially a
female institution: the lore of family and family culture itself—stories,
rituals, traditions, icons, sayings—are preserved and promulgated primarily
by women" (p. 19). At the same time, Carolyn Heilbrun argues from her
analysis of women's biographies and autobiographies that "women have

been deprived of the narratives, or the texts, plots, or examples, by which they might assume power over—take control of—their own lives" (1988, p. 17). Of prime importance is thus "woman's quest for her own story" (p. 17). As Joanne Frye echoes, "men have told the stories and framed the cultural precepts; women, reading those stories and bound by those precepts, have too often found themselves living men's stories rather than telling and living their own" (1986, p. i).

Despite the apparent disagreement between these two perspectives, gender studies generally have spawned a family of foundational questions that haunt any consideration of the storied nature of human life. For example, do women tell—and write—their lifestories in essentially different ways from those of men? Do they live out significantly different life-plots, and subscribe to markedly different ways of characterizing themselves in the midst of their life's events? Besides obvious individual differences, are there fundamental *gender* differences in how people remember, how they talk about themselves and listen to others (Tannen, 1990), and how they make sense of their experience? Such questions are so basic and big that we would be deluding ourselves if we presumed that, as two men, we could deal with them adequately in what follows. Nonetheless, we have tried to acknowledge them wherever relevant to our perspective.

Wide as this survey seems, it far from exhausts the many works in which the story model plays a central role. It also refers to several issues on which we certainly have an opinion but to which, like the gender ones just mentioned, we cannot give thorough treatment. Among these is a tangle of issues concerning the intricate relationship between language, time, and narrative that are presently being debated on the complex frontier where literary theory intersects with psychoanalytic theory, cultural studies, cognitive science, and linguistic analysis.

Another set of issues has to do with human memory. Insofar as memory is our subject in this book, we deal with it not in a technical or empirical manner but in terms of the metaphor of life as story. Accordingly, we make little attempt to cross-reference our perspective with distinctions commonly employed to penetrate the mystery of this faculty, such as episodic and semantic memory, explicit and implicit memory, voluntary and involuntary memory, long- and short-term memory, body memory, and so on (see Schachter, 1996). If one such distinction is our focus, however, it is the all-embracing memory that a cadre of theorists are starting to study: *autobiographical memory.*

Autobiographical memory is memory for "a whole life-time" and is decidedly personal (as opposed to procedural) in nature. It is "the sum of

[our] knowledge of [our] own lives and as such is the basis for a concept of self" (Rubin, 1986, p. 69). Our interest here is in the narrative, even fictional, dimensions of such memory and the changes that occur in both its content and form over the course of the lifespan. However, because this book is looking at autobiographical *reflection*, or thinking, it is not only memory—not solely our sense of the past—with which we are concerned but our sense of the future as well, our *pro*-flection: the dynamics of anticipation and expectation as much as of remembering and reminiscence. In other words, storying our lives—like re-storying them—is not a past-oriented process alone, anymore than is the process of writing, and reading, a novel.

Despite these limits to the scope of what follows, this survey underlines not only the narrative complexity of everyday life, but also the importance of storytelling per se, a practice as ancient as language itself. Interest in story thus draws on a history far longer than that of current, often esoteric "discourse" on the narrative question. Moreover, as we shall see throughout, free use of the story metaphor has implications for our analyses of all aspects of the human enterprise—not just our abstract theories on human nature but also our understanding of deep change in our own and others' lives, and of the ethics that guide our conduct in everyday ways. Finally, this survey underscores the dubiousness of any treatment of lifestory that restricts itself to one field alone. In order to explore the storying and restorying of our lives we must travel through interdisciplinary territory all the way, a fact that makes the adventure ahead of us as daunting as it surely is enticing.

THE NEED FOR PERSONAL STORYTELLING

We often hear these days that we are living in an information age, a digital world, a global village, or a postmodern society. This transition, it is argued, reflects a major shift from a more stable modern society in which people had larger myths or grand narratives with which they could identify and on the basis of which they could live. First, for example, we hear that we could rely more on traditional family structures, whereas now we have high divorce rates, many single parents, children with two sets of parents, children raised by grandparents, and so on. A second grand narrative that is said to be obsolete or ineffective as a story to live by is work. We hear that people will have work but no jobs. Downsizing or rightsizing is a hallmark of current postmodern society. Loyalty and a mutual relationship between employer and employee are disappearing.

Third, we hear that many people are disillusioned with organized religion and more focused on a materialistic or this-world lifestory. The grand narrative of finding our place in the world by identifying with the great religious stories has weakened considerably. Finally, people feel that their lives are managed or directed from the outside; that, in addition to public management of health, education, and work, their lives are divided into socially prescribed stages of childhood, adolescence, and adulthood.

The above scenario has prompted some to suggest that, in a postmodern world, our identity as persons amounts to little more than "a proliferation of shifting signs and meanings, rapidly changing images seemingly lacking enduring substance" (Gubrium, 1995, p. 5). A metaphor for this characterization is the MTV video self. Whether this metaphor is an effective one to describe ourselves today is an issue that will be debated as time goes on; however, it is clear that many people and societies are experiencing serious problems as a result of the fundamental changes in the themes and plots characterizing the stories of our lives as we approach the twenty-first century.

These problems stem from one apparent implication of postmodernism, which is a separatedness, or lack of relatedness, that has resulted in what gerontologists like Tom Cole (1992) and Harry Moody (1991) describe as a widespread sense of meaninglessness or a spiritual malaise. This feeling of separation occurs at at least three levels. First, for many people, "the story of my life" consists of a lack of meaning beyond the material. There is an exclusive emphasis on the *via activa,* or outer achievement and control aspects of our lifestory. Therefore, we are separate from our deeper inner nature as spiritual beings. Second, we are separate from that same social story since it is itself, as we described above, managed through social policy from the outside. We often feel powerless to influence the unfolding of the social story that, nevertheless, remains part of our identity. Third, we are separate in that we see our story as individual; this is sometimes called *privatism*. We identify ourselves as unique and apart from other persons; we have little sense of community or collective understanding of where we are going as human beings, and of the meaning of aging. The meaning of life becomes the meaning of *my* life as a unique individual. Unfortunately, this is a plot, or theme, that often gains ascendance in times of scarce resources; that is, many people become very territorial and "circle the wagons."

In this book, we explore the many ways in which a focus on the metaphor of life as story can contribute to a positive and meaningful interpretation of the postmodern dilemma we have just described. In other words, that dilemma, though accurate, troublesome, and commonly observed, is not the only possible outcome—or *story*—of the information society. Rather, the movement away from traditional grand narratives may lead us to explore and personalize our own stories and our own world. In fact, some of us may find an even deeper meaning in those same narratives, yet move beyond blind adherence to one in particular.

METAPHORS

One of the basic assumptions of this volume is that we not only *have* stories but *are* stories. A corollary of this view is that all language is metaphorical, or storied. Besides the common metaphors of "the mind as a computer" or "human beings as machines," examples can be found in various therapeutic approaches. Each is based on a set of metaphors, as indicated by Freud's use of sexual symbolism as a way of decoding dreams and fantasies; or Jung's creation of the notions of "animus" and "anima" as a way of understanding basic forces in human nature; or humanistic psychologists' talk about "peak experiences" and behaviorists' about "little black boxes" (Schroots et al., 1991). In the same vein, we can point to the metaphorical basis of scientific theories and of religious beliefs . In relation to the latter, in fact, the activity of hermeneutics has arisen—that is, the science of interpretation, specifically of biblical texts. As it is, then, we bring a storied perspective to a variety of metaphors. However, our focus here is on the story metaphor itself and on the implications of its entailments—plot, character, setting, genre, and point of view—for our own lives.

In essence, we are engaging in what the philosopher Hans Gadamer (1976) calls *philosophical hermeneutics*, which is a process of recovering the meaning in something we have come to take for granted. The reason this is so important to do, for research, practice, and everyday life, is that there are root metaphors—or metaphors integral to a particular theory, approach, or view of ourselves—that are often implicit, but which, over time, become dogma-like and get embraced with something like religious zeal. They develop an immune system (Bridges, 1980). Though originally created to guide thinking and practice toward some other end, such as understanding a particular aspect of human nature, they come to define a person or condition right from the outset. For example, you are diagnosed as having these symptoms, therefore you must be a certain way. Witness the stereotypical statement uttered when, as an adult, you visit your doctor: "What do you expect at your age?!"

To paraphrase a Zen Buddhist saying, this is a case of mistaking the finger pointing at the moon for the moon itself. However, a focus on stories assists us in the critical process of making implicit metaphors explicit, permitting us to assess them on their own merits and in terms of their appropriateness to understanding the particular biographical encounter in which we find ourselves, again, in research, practice, or everyday life. As Gubrium (1995, p. 12) puts it, "while programs to teach active listening are packaged and sold by the therapeutic culture industry, what it means in practice to be an active listener is articulated locally in relation to biographical particulars."

Throughout this book, we thus emphasize topics like storylistening in order to demonstrate the need for a continuous return to the voice of the other. Our hope is to contribute to the process of disentangling our own personal and professional story from that of the person to whom we are listening, so far as that is possible. In fact, we shall see in the coming chapters just how all these dimensions are involved in any biographical encounter. To repeat, the key to effective storylistening is to listen to all of the constituent dimensions, or voices, in the story the person tells. This is clearly a process, and sometimes not an obvious or simple one, for we do not always easily let go of our favorite metaphors, myths, or images, particularly if they have been professionally sanctioned.

Another important point in this context is that, from a metaphorical or storied perspective, there is no such thing as *the* truth or *the* true story, apart from a particular context or biographical encounter. This is what is referred to as the "hermeneutic circle": There is no such thing as an objective truth that can be read from a static reality that exists outside that circle. "Truth" thus becomes a search for the best fit between story and person. As we discuss frequently in what follows, a therapist, teacher, or parent—in other words, a storylistener—is not in the business of being an expert in someone else's life. Rather than script-writers of that person's story, they are *coauthors*. Following Gadamer (1976) again, while I cannot totally separate my metaphors, my story, or my "preunderstandings" from yours, I can attempt to distinguish between blind, or unreflected, preunderstandings and ones that are enabling, in the sense of allowing you to create your own story. From this perspective, therefore, there is a moral dimension to truth and knowledge, in that we are called to *dialogue*, with an intention to seek the truth, not to *rhetoric*, with an intention to coerce another person to accept "my" truth.

CONCLUSION

Our purpose in this chapter has been to introduce you to the basic themes or assumptions of *our* story of the life as story metaphor. We have also provided an introduction to some of the larger issues—to the larger story—

our perspective lives within. This larger story includes the intense interest in storying in various disciplines in the humanities and social sciences, as well as in areas of practice or intervention. After viewing just a sampling of this larger story, we hope you will see that the story metaphor is rich, complex, multifaceted, and worthy of serious study. However, we invite you now to join us in a process of serious "play," as we proceed to consider some important theoretical issues involved in the restorying of our lives.

Chapter 2

Understanding the Story Metaphor: Theoretical Issues

> When it comes to finding a new mythology, a new guiding truth, that can fill the void around us—that can be a myth, a truth, we can live with—the first place to turn is our own story, our own truth, our own spirituality, our own search for meaning.
>
> Robert Atkinson (1995)

INTRODUCTION

Not only do we *have* a lifestory, but we *are* stories: This statement captures the basic importance of lifestories and personal storytelling. It means that our very experience can be characterized from a story perspective. That is, stories are cognitive: they contain ideas. They are affective: they involve emotions. And they are volitional: they involve activity or behavior. Our thoughts, feelings, and actions, even our personal identity, can thus be understood as a story. This means that life as story is what philosophers call an ontological metaphor; it is basic to who we are as human beings. The term ontology comes from "ontos" or being, which means what is, and "logos," which means story or account. Therefore, ontology is the story of what is. There are many possible ontologies, including the major religious and cultural stories of the universe and our place in it.

As an ontological metaphor, life as story can be contrasted with other scientific and professional metaphors, such as the stimulus-response perspective of behaviorism, or the bundle of social roles metaphor contained in particular sociological theories, or the postmodern version of the self that we introduced in Chapter 1. From these perspectives, the notion of personal storytelling is seen to be either the result of, on the one hand, various bio-psycho-behavioral reactions over the lifespan, or, on the other hand, the result of sociocultural conditioning. In both of these cases, the story of my life is not really mine in the sense that I do not participate in the creation of that story; rather, I am carried along by outside forces and constraints. Thus, common statements such as "my genes made me do it" or "society made me do it." Finally, in Chapter 1 we discussed the MTV video self that has no real center.

Nevertheless, at another extreme, it is inaccurate to say that somehow we each have a totally unique lifestory that we create in a spiritual, individual vacuum, that is, completely from the inside, and by which we are able to function in life without being affected by the physical, psychological, and social dimensions of human nature. The solution to this dilemma comes by way of a closer look at the elements of the life as story metaphor. Though we take up a more detailed analysis of it in Chapter 3, an overview at this point will set the stage for our basic orientation in this volume.

DIMENSIONS OF LIFESTORIES

It is possible to identify at least four interrelated dimensions of our lifestories. First, there is our *structural* story, which includes such things as social policy and power relations in a society. Structural constraints can effectively silence personal stories or voices, as evidenced in programs and associated attitudes that systematically discriminate against, for example, older persons (ageism and mandatory retirement) or women (sexism and pay equity). Second, there is our *social* story, or the social meanings associated with storytelling, including such relationships as professional and client, or employer and, in an aging postmodern society, younger and older workers. This dimension also includes ethnic and cultural aspects of lifestories. Third, there is our *interpersonal* story, which refers to relationships of intimacy, confidant or confidante, families, and love. Finally, there is the dimension of personal meaning or our *personal* story itself. This is the dimension consisting of the creation and discovery of our life history or herstory, the way in which the pieces make or do not make sense to a person.

In the following chapters, we will be exploring the many ways in which these dimensions of our stories influence each other and how they together make up the stories we are. You may find this a useful framework to look at your own story or that of another in terms of both identifying the sources of your story—structural, social, and so on—and noting how these influences change and can be changed over the lifespan. An example would be an older widow who finally becomes her personal story as a business person, after a life dominated by structural and social obligations to her family and her spouse. Or the retired engineer who becomes an artist after having been prevented from expressing his personal dimension by a rigid social and parental story, and then having had to forego this story again as a younger man to be a single parent. It is fascinating simply to listen to a lifestory with these four dimensions in mind, and with no judgment attached to that listening, but rather just being open to the emerging themes.

In contrast to the video version of postmodernism described earlier, the personal dimension of our story is operative in ordinary life, and stories are lived even while philosophical crises arrive and depart (Gubrium, 1995). More than ever before in history, with the demise of grand cultural narratives, people may have to rely on their own biography (Mader, 1991, 1996), opportunities for restorying, and their cultivated sense of possibility. Thus, far from not having a self or a personal, inside story, this aspect of our nature is becoming more center stage.

The foregoing outline highlights the complexity and richness of the story metaphor. While many dimensions go to make up lifestories, the bottom line of the life as story metaphor is that stories ultimately have to do with what is personal and what is meaningful. It is the characteristic of personal meaning that distinguishes the story metaphor from many other theories of human nature and makes it an effective metaphor for the study of human development.

But what do we mean by "meaning" and by "personal"? At first glance, speaking about personal meaning appears to contradict what we just said about the many other and outside components of our stories. That is, if lifestories are ultimately personal, then we can make up any story we want that suits our fancy; and if they are not personal in this sense, then the story is being constructed for us and the meaning it has for us is also determined from outside.

We find an answer to this problem by referring to the existentialist insight that human beings live in situations or contexts. And, human beings are always going beyond themselves by attempting to attribute a significance to those situations. In other words, people are constantly learning from and being influenced by the physical and human environment in which they find themselves located. As the philosopher Maurice Merleau-Ponty would say, in this way, human beings are involved in a process of creating and being created at the same time (Kenyon, 1988). Another way to say this is that persons are not self-enclosed individuals, or that the biographical unit does not correspond to the biological body. From this point of view, the challenge for ourselves, both personally and as researchers and practitioners, is to hold the various dimensions of lifestories in mind at the same time, and to resist the temptation to prematurely reduce a storied being to one dimension or another.

We have said that creating and discovering meaning in situations is a basic feature of being human. To take the discussion one step further, there is a fundamental connection between that meaning-giving activity and biography or storytelling. In fact, one could characterize human situations or contexts as *biographical encounters*, and the various dimensions of lifestories as *biographizers*, as the German psychoanalyst Wilhelm Mader (1996) terms them. The point here is that what people find meaningful about themselves and their world is made manifest or expressed through language in the form of metaphors and narratives or stories. To quote David Carr, "There is nothing below this narrative structure, at least nothing experienceable by us or comprehensible in experiential terms" (1986, p. 66). Or, as other authors have stated, stories are lived before they are told. Further, from this point of view, there is no literal reality, say, made up of information processing chips, which we then make into stories, for better or worse, so to speak. On the contrary, stories are the very stuff of human experience and the chips are themselves characters in a particular scientific story. This is what we referred to in Chapter 1 as the hermeneutic circle and the idea that there is no objective truth outside this intersubjective context.

Thus, whether we are concerned with science, practice, or everyday life, narratives and stories *are* the way the world is for us; they represent human reality, reality as it is for beings who live in situations or contexts, and who are self-creating in that context. Literary narratives are to be seen as more self-conscious and technical renderings of experience. Such a view is in contrast with the idea that narratives and lifestories impose on events a form that they themselves do not have. Stories from this viewpoint become window dressing or something incidental to real knowledge. Personal storytelling represents such things as wishful thinking, an escape from reality, or perhaps spinning one's wheels.

The view that storytelling is unimportant or even a sign of pathology was widespread in gerontological research and practice until some fifteen years ago, and is still believed by some. Falling into this category, for example, is the idea of employing any form of reality therapy with dementing persons, as opposed to providing them the opportunity to tell their stories in any way they can, and more importantly, listening to those stories. The ethical issues that arise in this regard will be discussed in Chapter 6. However, part of the reason for the lack of significance given to storytelling concerns a particular view of time and aging.

CLOCK TIME AND STORYTIME

As we have just mentioned, until recently, there was a powerful stereo-type operating in both professional circles and the general public, that such things as reminiscence and storytelling were to be viewed as signs of pathology or senility. Moreover, it was often thought that psychological and psychodynamic intervention with older persons was a waste of time as people's personalities were already "locked in." In contrast to this, today there is a large interest in such areas as geropsychiatry and various forms of practice directed to counseling and therapy with older persons. Further, from the perspective being elaborated here, storytelling and stories are an integral aspect of identity and meaning in life at any age.

One aspect of this development has to do with the way in which we understand and, more importantly, *live* time as human beings. In fact, one could claim that gerontologists are among those who are contributing to a new perspective on time, one that reflects more the assumptions of an Einsteinian universe than of a Newtonian one. In everyday terms what this means is that we are moving from a view in which past, present, and future are linear and separate to a view in which they are connected and interrelated. One way to show this is by way of the distinction between outer time-aging and inner time-aging.

Outer Time-Aging

Outer time-aging refers to calendar time, clock time, and social time or social clocks. Social gerontologists have claimed that people judge themselves to be on-time or off-time with respect to major life-course issues such as career, marriage, and family. This view often gives the impression that our lives are determined or locked in by earlier experiences. Human life is measured in terms of chronological time and the social meanings that are attached to clock time. Life becomes a straight line and we are determined by a static or rigid past and a future that is daily becoming of increasingly short duration. As Plank (1989, p. 33) explains:

We commonly accept this essentialistic view of the past as a thing or a series of events which happened once and for all in a specific way and which we, as historians, as witnesses in court, or merely as ordinary men who must live with what they have done, can grasp by a careful perusal of our memories or appropriate archives and documents.

Is it possible that this view of time and aging is itself a story and, as such, something we have created individually and culturally and then decided to continue to believe?

Inner Time-Aging

In contrast to outer time-aging, a close look at lifestories highlights the insight that there is also an inner time-aging. For example, as Simone de Beauvoir (1973, p. 420) has noted, "Our private inward experience does not tell us the number of our years; no fresh perception comes into being to show us the decline of age." This means that aging and the experience of time is as much an inside personal story as it is an outside social story. Further, this view suggests that we can do something about the story of our own time and aging, if it tends to be one that reflects negative stereotypes that we buy into from the often powerful outside story. As Birren (1987) says, we can trade in and trade up our personal metaphors of aging. The interesting feature of this view becomes the creative ways in which people interact with the outer clock, which, even if it does not determine our being, must be dealt with as part of the larger story we live within.

Let us explore a little further the nature of inner time-aging as it can be seen in lifestories. Particularly in the case of older persons, storytelling does involve a considerable past dimension, a past life, including patterns of meaning or plots constructed earlier on. However, that past is being reconstructed in serving the present. Today's story uses present, and therefore, in a sense, new, metaphors or storylines about past events. As C. S. Lewis has noted, "I never expected to have, in my sixties, the happiness that passed me by in my twenties" (Atkinson, 1995, p. 76). What this means is that a person does not exist in the past; the past exists in a person. Even very old people, although they must adjust to the limited number of years left to them in outer time-aging terms, are still *living* time with a present, past, and future. Joyce Horner (1982, p. 16) describes the situation in this way, in referring to her fellow nursing home resident: "I don't think anyone old is *afraid* of death, though many, including Mrs. B., who will be 108 on Monday, may want life to go on." It would seem that so long as we are alive, we still have a story to tell and we still have a past, present, and future.

And yet, a focus on *biographical aging* (Kenyon, 1996a) indicates that just because we are stories does not imply that we always want to tell that story or that we should encourage everyone to engage in storytelling so that they can, say, die peacefully, or be psychosocially competent in their later years. This view was evident in some earlier writings on the use of approaches like *life review*, such as those by Robert Butler (1963). The idea here was that all older persons would desire to review their lives or tell their stories, due to approaching death. Thus, the claim is that people would want to tie up their life or bring things to a resolution before they die.

This claim has been subjected to various criticisms, the main one being that, although it is a biographical approach, it really buys into an outer time-aging perspective, in at least two ways. First, being older does not guarantee that someone will become aware of their finitude in some explicit way that will make them need to tell their story. A number of researchers, including Webster (1994), have reported that the desire to reminisce or review one's life is not necessarily tied to age, and that expected triggers of reminiscence such as approaching death are not always evident. And second, this view assumes that the prospect of death in later life makes one lose a sense of the future or a future perspective. Our discussion of inner time-aging suggests that this does not fully reflect the way in which we can experience time.

A further criticism of this perspective concerns whether, as storied beings, it is true that we always can or even desire to tie everything up in our lives, in order to have a good death. Gubrium (1993, p. 188) makes this point effectively in the following way:

The longitudinal material gathered from residents interviewed more than once indicates that the very idea of a course of adjustment at the end of life shortchanges its variety, complexity, improvisations. There is little overall evidence that affairs are ultimately settled, sundered ties finally repaired, transgressions at last righted or accounted for, or preparations for the future or afterlife completed. While some residents, of course, do speak of waiting for heaven, buying cemetery plots, and making funeral arrangements—points of information that indeed may hold considerable value for them—these do not necessarily signify terminal horizons.

BASIC LIFESTORY QUESTIONS

There are significant ethical issues associated with Gubrium's observations which we will address in Chapter 6. In the meantime, there are four important aspects of lifestories that follow from its existential or human foundation. These aspects, discussed here from a theoretical perspective, raise crucial questions, questions that constitute underlying themes throughout this volume.

Transparency: Are Lifestories Totally Visible?

Because we are always in this situation and not another, our stories are stories from a particular point of view. And, more than this, that point of view changes with time, new experiences, and even the very telling of our story. There is, therefore, a characteristic of *opacity* associated with life-stories. It is like seeing through a glass darkly. This means that we cannot and do not see all or know all there is to know, about ourselves, other people, or the world.

Completeness: Can We Ever Have the Whole Story?

We can never understand exhaustively our own lifestory or that of another person, since no story is ever complete. There are three ways to show that this is the case. First, as we just noted, when I look at your story, it is from my point of view, which is only one among many other points of view. In this sense, each of us is unique and each has a personal, inside story. Even though we can, at the same time, listen to, understand, and communicate our stories, it is not possible ever to arrive at the final truth, the whole truth, and nothing but the truth about a life. The station-stops on our journeys may be similar (Kenyon, 1991), but our stories are never exactly alike.

Second, when I look at my own story, I am in the middle of it as I look at it. I am stopping the story to look at it, but my life as story goes on as a continuous process. As Donald Polkinghorne (1988, p. 150) notes: "We are in the middle of our stories and cannot be sure how they will end; we are constantly having to revise the plot as new events are added to our lives." In this sense, then, neither an autobiography nor a biography is ever complete.

Third, we could go so far as to say that not even death, which may end a life, brings an end to a lifestory that lives on in other persons and or in a culture. In fact, as writers such as Gabriel Marcel (Kenyon, 1980) and Victor Frankl (1962), among others, have discussed, a person's lifestory may continue to live on in a very real way through a loved one after death.

Coherence: Are We One Story or Many?

Although in one sense we can say that I have *a* lifestory, in reality it is difficult to discover exactly what that story is. We seem to be many stories at once, and although these many stories all belong to me, they may not add up to one recognizable and integrated version of *the* story of my life. As you will hear in Chapters 3 and 4, and as already pointed to, we are social stories, interpersonal stories, economic stories, ethnic stories, among others, all at once. It is for this reason that David Carr (1986) has expressed the sentiment that a detailed biography does not necessarily make a good story.

It is possible that we are many stories in another sense. Over time, we live stories that we do not blend together easily into an overall meaning or coherence—for example, in the case of divorce or the loss of a significant other, followed by remarriage, or in the case of a basic career change. As we proceed, an interesting question here is whether these many partial lifestories need ever fit into one overarching narrative with a neat beginning, middle, and end.

Support for the idea that we are many stories also comes from looking at research that is increasingly showing that people do not have ready-made lifestories that they express when asked to "just tell your story." Rather, stories seem to emerge from the situation or the biographical encounter. In other words, what we emphasize, what we find in storytelling, depends on who is asking and why. An interesting example of research in this area is the work of photographer Joanne Leonard (1994). In her studies of what she calls photographic meaning, female identity, family, and layered auto-biographical storytelling, Leonard notes that, "I'm interested in non-linear narratives: disjointed, multi-voiced, ambiguous as is memory and impossibly positioned in time, a narrative that resists 'sentencing.' Photographs, like memories, are ambiguous; their stories usually remain unclear, merely hinted at" (p. 657). There is a refusal here to represent lifestories as if they can be reduced to a single coherent narrative, and thereby be objectified, which risks their losing their aliveness. The issue of whether and in what ways we can say that we are one story or many is complex and open to further debate. The "many" story argument is presented here with some of its implications and the "one" story argument appears in Chapter 3.

Adequacy: Will Just Any Story Do?

From the fact that we are many stories, does it follow that we tell ourselves and others different stories to suit the situation? Are all lifestories lies? The idea of many stories can be clarified by looking again at the fact that we are stories, but stories from a point of view. This does not mean, however, that to change a point of view means changing our story completely to suit the audience, so to speak. Rather, it indicates that we are indeed creating meaning in a particular situation, a situation that is already larger than we as individuals.

As we will see in Chapter 5, we are only coauthors of our stories. So, although we are involved creatively in the content of our stories, this does not mean that we can become any story we want or change the plot at will. We are free to make ourselves, but not to make ourselves *up*. To repeat, this is because our personal story is influenced by the structural, social, and interpersonal dimensions we discussed earlier. The paradox here is that "I" have a crucial role to play in making my own story meaningful in a "we" situation, made up of other people, a culture, and a physical environment.

Following the philosopher Jean-Paul Sartre, our stories are made up of two components. The first is called *facticity*, which comes from the outside, reflects what we will discuss in Chapter 4 as "the larger story we live within," and includes the story we tell ourselves or buy into at any moment. However, second, stories also contain a sense of *possibility*, which means choices or new meanings. As Maddi (1988, p. 183) explains: "Our sense of what is possible is intertwined with what we perceive as given, and the dynamic balance between the two gives our lives its particular flavor." This feature of life as story suggests grounds for optimism concerning potentially positive directions for our future in that, from a storied point of view, it is not clear, up front, which parts of our stories and ourselves are locked in by facticity and which parts are open to being traded in and traded up, or open to possibility. We will be considering some interesting ideas on this topic in the following chapters.

TRUTH, LIES, AND STORYTELLING

But what about the question whether lifestories are simply lies fabricated to give someone what they want to hear? Is there such a thing as "the truth, the whole truth, and nothing but the truth?" From the point of view of life as story, as we pointed out in Chapter 1, all language is metaphorically based, and thus the notion of truth or authenticity is situational or relative to a context. Here we again encounter the hermeneutic circle. What this means is that in some situations we can take a person's story at face value; the story is the truth for him or her and reflects the way in which he or she finds meaning. There need be no further assessment of that story in order for us to understand that person or even to facilitate a higher quality of life. As Jaber Gubrium (1993, p. 15) points out in discussing nursing home residents he studied, "The life narratives in this book should be read, accordingly, not in terms of whether, say, Jake Bellows actually was a stand-up comic on the road fifty weeks of the year, but in terms of how he links that experience to his feeling of being 'at home' in the nursing facility, his way of conveying subjective meaning." Or, as George Fowler (1995, p. 25) points out in his autobiography, *Dance of a Fallen Monk*, "whether or not Grandmother Fowler was actually the tyrant my father remembered is not so important as the fact that that is how he carried her memory, like burning acid, in his heart."

In other cases, for example, when stories are used in a geriatric assessment context, there is usually a need to go beyond the patient's story in order to corroborate the information disclosed and to seek additional details from medical records, the person's family, and so on. The idea that truth is related to a context also applies to biographical forms of research. Again, the extent to which one looks at data—in this case, lifestories—depends on the purpose of the study. One can never know the whole truth about a person, but that is not necessarily a problem. It is a feature of being human, which means that we always have something to learn (for a further discussion of the use of lifestories in research, see Ruth and Kenyon, 1996).

POTENTIAL PERSONAL CHANGE AND GROWTH THROUGH STORIES

In the following chapters, we explore in more detail the "how" of personal storytelling and restorying. In other words, we are concerned with the ways in which it may be possible to transcend our facticity and expand our sense of possibility. However, prior to this, it is necessary to indicate some further theoretical issues regarding life as story that deal with the possibility of growth through stories. Of relevance here is the following admission by Randall (1995, p. 16) concerning his work in the area of counseling, "I found it difficult not to feel that if only we are offered a hospitable space in which we can tell and re-tell our story however we wish, then, through the storytelling process itself, we open ourselves to whatever measure of clarification or healing for which we happen to be ready at the time."

Although this statement reflects the basic assumption of this volume, namely, that everyone is a story and that we are all meaning-seekers or learners through stories, we need to revisit some of the dimensions of this process. While some of the following remarks apply to other groups and issues, a focus on our aging society and world can serve as an example.

Restorying in an Aging Society

Aging or an Overemployed Plot

It is the case that many older persons subscribe to negative stereotypes and images of aging, even though we pointed out earlier that there is an inner aging or an inside story about aging that does not correspond to this outer perspective. This means that people do not necessarily become old from the inside. Rather, through pressures to conform or due to the lack of an opportunity to explore their sense of possibility, they are working with outdated or negative metaphors, or in terms of old stories: old in time and old in reference to themselves.

Prado (1986) has suggested that as we grow older we find particular narratives or, as we say in Chapter 3, *signature stories* to be very effective as we go about our lives. However, this reliance on particular stories can lead to *perspective narrowing* and might result in what looks like rigidity or an inability to learn. The problem here is that the past effectiveness of particular stories or personal metaphors can prevent us from searching for new images and plots, even when the circumstances of both the traveler and the voyage have changed (Kenyon, 1991). It is important to notice that from this point of view aging does not reflect some kind of inevitable, encroaching personality rigidity. Rather, it reflects a situation in which a story has been told and a plot refined to the point of counterproductiveness. Therefore, what is needed here, and what can be provided through storytelling, is access to new stories, new meanings, or new wrinkles in established patterns.

Storytelling in an Ageist Society

From what we have just said, the story perspective can be seen to provide a potentially optimistic direction for lifelong learning and positive aging. However, we should not minimize the constraints to what is possible in biographical aging. In the western world, it is still the case that we live in a culture that both explicitly and implicitly discriminates against older persons. Practices such as mandatory retirement, whether formal or simply the result of the "empty desk syndrome," inappropriate institutionalization, and paternalistic social policy—the "we know what is best for you" syndrome— all these result in a situation in which an older person's inside story is severely challenged by their outside story—a sad story for many.

Under these conditions it is not difficult to understand why many older people simply resign themselves to an outer image of aging, and existing *storyotypes*, or even continue to work with plots from the past, whether or not they really work today. This makes sense since they cannot maintain an open relationship between the person they are inside, their inside story, and the social and structural dimensions of their story, the outside story.

It needs to be repeated that this state of affairs is not the result of biological decline with age—that is, not something natural and inevitable. It is the result of a particular set of social circumstances. Nevertheless, it is an important issue since it places many older persons at risk. Mader (1991), for example, indicates that older persons are increasingly at risk of such things as pathological narcissism. This basically means that people close in upon themselves in an unhealthy manner as a result of the combination of, on the one hand, various losses associated with aging, including those that concern the body, work, significant others, and even the self, and, on the other hand, the lack of new meaningful self-images that can be expressed and given support in the older person's lived experiences. Another way to say this is that, in this situation, there is too much facticity and too little possibility. Nevertheless, it is not the aging process itself that is responsible for this state of affairs.

Aging constitutes only one of many examples that can be provided of contexts where an investigation of the dynamics of storytelling in postmodern society is crucial. Others that could be explored include feminist issues and ethnic and racial issues. However, a detailed look at these stories is beyond the scope of this volume.

What Is Possible in Storytelling

In postmodern western society, opportunities for storytelling do not often occur naturally, and it is not commonplace for a person to take the time to listen and tell one's story to oneself or to another, to reflect on one's aging and life. In contrast, what is being advocated here is that storytelling is basic to human nature; it is an existential or spiritual phenomenon due to its intimate connection to meaning. But if we grant this idea, what do we see in stories or from a storied perspective? How do they contribute to personal growth? In what follows, we shall provide an overview of the contribution and some features of life as story. These issues are then taken up in more detail in other chapters.

Gaining a Perspective on Our Lives or Getting the Story Out

The very *perceptual turn* of viewing our life as story leads to a detachment or breathing space between us and our story. This basic movement can enhance personal meaning by providing an opportunity for newness. Through this process we can give ourselves a break and allow our sense of possibility to come to the fore. We can utilize our imagination in the service of our own lives. This does not mean that we all must find a good therapist. In some cases, this is the appropriate modality; however, for most people, what is required is an unstructured or minimally structured, but supportive and nonjudgmental environment. We need more approaches that encourage people to find their own directions. The actual process of getting the story out is discussed in Chapter 5.

Good Stories and Meaningful Lives

Personal storytelling can help people to experience a basic acceptance of their lives, or to *own* their lives, as Florida Scott-Maxwell (1968) has said. However, this basic acceptance may take many forms, and it is important to clarify what we can expect with respect to our own lifestory, and in listening to the stories of others, either as professionals or friends. If it is true that our stories are partly visible and partly invisible to us, that they lack completeness at least in an existential sense, and that we may be multiple stories, then given these human dimensions, we can ask whether our lives must be capable of being configured into a well-written story with a good beginning, middle, and end, in order for us to find meaning. Do all the pieces need to fit in the end? It is at this point where it is crucial to make some distinctions between human life and the story metaphor.

In discussing this issue, the work of Erik Erikson (1963) is a common reference. Some interpretations of his work suggest that his last stage of human development, ego integrity versus despair, describes a situation in which a person must have a truly coherent lifestory in order to achieve meaning and wisdom and die having lived a full life. If not, older age is a time of despair and regret.

The important point here is that, if taken literally, this perspective does not reflect the existential-spiritual dimensions of human storytelling and human development. While we are claiming that we are stories and, as such, all is not chaos, it is not necessarily the case that we are one grand detailed narrative or that we can express what it is exactly that gives our life meaning. With respect to the first point, if we are stories, and we are always seeking meaning, then there must be some degree of coherence in the way that we go about the world. As David Carr (1986, p. 97) notes, "Things need to make sense. We feel the lack of sense when it goes missing."

However, as we will consider further in Chapter 6, the way that things make sense and the degree to which a life makes sense is another question. Some people are capable of marvelous articulation of their lifestory, and we find listening to or reading about their life an inspiring and pleasant experience. However, at the other extreme we might say that dementing persons are still telling and living a story that we can listen to in other ways. For example, a dementing person's emotional story may continue while his or her cognitive story appears to have ended. A further example would be the response of many people whom we would say accept their lives as we observe them and yet they may simply say something like "it was real." When it comes to stories, we might say that, on the one hand, the examined life is worth living; however, on the other hand, we can repeat David Carr's insight that a detailed biography does not necessarily make a good story.

This issue has to do with the second point we have just discussed regarding the completeness of a life. Some authors argue that good lives and good stories are both presumed to have a beginning, a middle, and a definite ending. It is true that our lifestory has a beginning, although, if we look at our evolutionary past, it is not clear where that beginning is located (Randall, 1995). It definitely has a middle in the sense of action or experience which is only partially tied to age or clock time. And, there is a definite end in physical death. But from a storied point of view, these designations become somewhat indefinite. People live on in others' stories; moreover, many people believe that our lifestory continues after death. And, in addition to these ideas, as Gubrium indicated earlier, there may be little evidence that people actually bring closure to their lifestory in any comprehensive manner in later life. Thus, we can ask: Does the human story ever really end?

LIFE AS STORY AND LIFE AS JOURNEY

The idea that our identity is formed on the basis of a story has the fundamental implication that we *become* the stories that we tell ourselves and the stories that we sometimes must live without our having explicitly consented to the plot. For example, we have looked at the notion of biographical aging as an attempt to understand how many persons buy into negative stereotypes of aging, imposed from the outside, and conversely, how many other older persons live stories that are meaningful and positive and perhaps express the wisdom of age. As such, the story metaphor contains tremendous potential for positive change and for finding meaning in a life, through both storytelling and, equally important, storylistening.

An effective way to summarize this chapter and to highlight the existential-spiritual ground out of which we live our stories is to appeal to the metaphor of the journey. Just as we previously posed four basic lifestory questions, here we can discuss four aspects of the journey metaphor that can provide a suggestive context for further dialogue concerning life as story, and its potential for facilitating personal growth.

1. The human journey is *personal*. There is an inviolable, unique, and intimate center to each of us, an inside story, which is not available to another and which is the source of personal meaning per se.

2. At the same time, our journey and story is social or *interpersonal*; the traveler is not alone or isolated by nature. In addition, the journey suggests possible experiences of wonder, anticipation, and curiosity, even though other negative experiences are also possible and even common. Relationships on the journey can range from Gabriel Marcel's (1962) ideas of presence, love, and communion, to the famous dictum by Jean-Paul Sartre (1955) in his earlier writings that "hell is other people."

3. The landscape of the journey resembles a winding path or a river rather than a prairie highway or a freeway. The traveler cannot know everything, neither in advance nor in hindsight. There are fundamental constraints to a panoramic vision most of the time; our view is opaque. This *opacity* brings with it elements of risk and chance, the necessity to choose among many paths, tributaries, or possible stories. Opacity also includes the fact that the stories may not all add up. In more literal terms, human beings are travelers who cannot always read off the truth about reality and life as a basis for appropriate action and decision-making.

4. The duration of the journey is indefinite and has an impermanent or *transitory* character. The fact of death makes the traveler finite; however, it is part of the opacity of the journey that we do not know when that part of the story will end. Further, we know that in some important ways, death does not end our story—that is, in our culture, and in the hearts of our loved ones. In these ways, the fellow traveler is still present, still telling a story, and still sharing our journey. Perhaps nothing really lasts except the journey itself, and we really are "en route." Perhaps it is the fact of death and impermanence that can provide the catalyst for either despair or wonder and openness, depending on the tale we are able to create and discover.

CONCLUSION

The journey constitutes an effective metaphor for characterizing life as story as we see it. However, other "genres" of stories are possible and will be discussed in the following chapters. The implication that a journey goes somewhere, that is, has a "telos" or end point, is also an important issue. We will consider some ideas about this topic in Chapter 7. As we proceed now to the next three chapters, the emphasis will move away from the theoretical and toward the practical. That is, we will look in detail, first, at the way that we are stories; second, at how we story our lives; and, third, at how we can restory our own lives and be agents of restorying for others.

Chapter 3

The Stories of Our Lives

A man is always a teller of tales; he lives surrounded by his stories and the stories of others; he sees everything that happens to him through them, and he tries to live his life as if he were recounting it.

Jean-Paul Sartre ([1938] 1965)

INTRODUCTION

Having considered the theoretical foundations of story as a metaphor for life, we are ready to try it on for size. We are ready to ask: just what do we mean by "the story of my life"? In this chapter, then, we get a feel for how many stories we actually carry around inside us, and how many *kinds* of stories. We also look at the *levels* on which the very notion of a lifestory can be understood. In general, we ponder "the fictional side of human nature" (Hillman, 1975, p. 128). In the next chapter, we consider where our stories come from—that is, why we have stories about these events and situations but not those, and have formed them in this manner but not that. In Chapter 5 we look at the implications of this formation process, especially as it changes over time. That is, we consider how our lives are continually being *re*-storied and, what is more, how we can direct that restorying and be agents of it in the lives of others.

For now, we want to focus not on story-*ing* or *re*-storying but simply the *stories* of our lives. First, we look at *The Stories Around Us*; then at *The Levels of Lifestory*; next at *The Library of Our Lives*. Finally, we consider the common conundrum of *One Event Yet Many Versions*, the concept of *The Novelty of Our Lives*, and the relationship between *Emotions and Stories*.

THE STORIES AROUND US

Before taking stock of the stories of our lives, we need to remind ourselves that an entire universe of stories lies around us already. We are "inescapably born into an already storied world" (Parry and Doan, 1994, p. 38). As we noted in Chapter 2 and shall see even more in the next chapter, we live our lifestories within a sociocultural context that is itself deeply storied from bottom to top, and is endlessly being *re*storied as well. True, we seldom sit by the campfire listening to our elders recite the old legends about the creation of the world or (sadly) relate what life was like when they and *their* elders were young. However, we delude ourselves if we think that storytelling as such is in danger of dying. Quite the contrary. To paraphrase the epigraph from Sartre at the start of this chapter, we live surrounded by our stories and the stories of others—stories of (or about) our neighbors, children, and colleagues, our lovers and friends. Besides the bombardment of jokes we all must endure, that is, we are immersed in a sea of *gossip* as well.

Whether we live in the countryside or the concrete canyons of the inner city, gossip abounds. Lip-smacking delight at learning what is the "truth" behind the events of the day is as much a part of life in the present as ever it was in the past, however different our ways of talking or the topics about which we talk. Indeed, gossip today has a higher profile than ever, with all the tabloids our hearts could desire detailing everything from the diets to the sex romps (real or concocted) of princes and politicians, musicians and movie stars. Tell-all autobiographies and biographical exposes—seldom have their sales been so strong, fired by our continuing lust for *the real story* we presume is behind the scenes.

As we go from print to screen, the numbers of stories only increase, with the typical TV able to funnel into our living rooms hour on hour of prefab fiction, from cartoons to sitcoms, and from two-hour miniseries to thirty-second morality plays plotting the conversions of consumers to the virtues of Brand X. And, should we get our fill of such stories, the corner store will be stocked with enough videotaped ones that it can take us half an evening to decide on the one to which, two nights out of seven, we shall probably treat ourselves.

Far from being dead, storytelling has scarcely been more alive. Journalists, politicians, preachers, producers, biographers, comedians, novelists, even scientists—everyone is spewing out stories continuously: about themselves, about others, about nature, about our world. Even the news has become synonomous with stories, and events are incipient tales, needing only the talent of a reporter to flesh them out and pass them on. If anything, the line between story and life is fuzzier than ever. And this, when the reign of science never seemed more solid, nor the border between fiction and fact better marked. With everyone's stories swirling so bewilderingly around us, it is little wonder that many of us feel we are losing touch with the richness of our own. Hence this book.

THE LEVELS OF LIFESTORY

The notion of a singular lifestory within which all our shorter stories have their home is both empowering and enchanting. We all believe we have such a lifestory and are only too happy to tell it, provided we have the right audience. Indeed, we take the very concept of "my life" to refer not to a set of statistics (about age, weight, or height) but to "my story." We also believe that everyone else has a lifestory too, and that if given an invitation, he or she will be tickled to recount it. As gerontology researcher John Kotre writes: "Though *life story* means many things to many people, it never fails to start words flowing. Despite scholarly arguments about what constitutes a story, no one has ever asked me what to do when beginning to relate his or her own" (1990, p. 26).

As Kotre suggests, however, the concept of a "lifestory" is far from clearcut. As to what exactly it *is*—"that's another story." Before we catalogue the material a lifestory may contain, then, the following detour should show why a definition is difficult to obtain. To help sort through the meanings we can attach to this everyday notion, there are at least four levels on which it can be understood: *outside, inside, inside-out,* and *outside-in.*

The Outside Story

First are the "unexpurgated" events of my *existence*, from conception to now: physical events, psychological events, biochemical events, even atomic ones. This is the level of "the bare facts," the vast sum of which *is* my story in a technical or objective sense. It is the reality of my life in the raw, however, because it is uninterpreted, unevaluated, and, in these respects, unexperienced. Thus, we can think of it as merely the *outside* story since, if knowable at all, it is only by some colossal computer at the edge of space-time.

The Inside Story

Second is what I *make* of these facts—or make *up* from them—within myself, subjectively. It is that portion of my existence that I have attended to and taken in, that I have made some sense of as it has flowed past me and through me. This level thus constitutes a different story from my outside one since it is merely a digest of the latter and ambiguously, sometimes contradictorily, related to it. A condition like hypochondria is an example. In reality, my health is fine; all the tests have come back negative. In my mind, however, the rash on my arm is the sure sign of cancer. My body tells me one story; my imagination, another. Furthermore, what makes it inside me (and so is available to my thoughts and feelings) is only a tiny proportion of what my existence actually entails. We need only think of the last long drive we took and the countless things our eyes observed and our senses registered en route, yet how little we could later recall when invited to talk about our trip.

Our life on this inside level is still vast, however, for it holds our memories of the past, our anticipations of the future, and, in the present, the mutterings of our mind and meanderings of our heart. "A penny for your thoughts?" pries a friend, wanting to get to know us better, and we can find the question galling, for our thoughts can be so many and can change so fast. In the space of seconds, our incessant self-chatter can be crammed by a dozen ideas, a swirl of half-formed hunches, and a host of feelings and recollections about the widest variety of matters. As put by novelist Thomas Wolfe (1983), all manner of "flicks and darts and haunting lights" can present themselves "unbidden at an unexpected moment: a voice once heard; an eye that looked; a mouth that smiled; a face that vanished; the way the sunlight came and went; the rustling of a leaf upon a bough; a stone, a leaf, a door" (p. 44). We can think of all of this as the story-*behind*-the story or the *inside* story, our private inner world—what can be called our *experience.* It is that swirling mass of "quasi-narrative" inner material (Casey, 1987) from which emerge our dreams (themselves generally storied) and which, to quote controversial psychiatrist, R. D. Laing, "used to be called the Soul" (1967, p. 18).

The Inside-Out Story

Third is the way I take this inside story, abridge it, and, wittingly or not, edit it for others—not only *telling* it with my words but *showing* it with my deeds. As psychoanalyst Roy Schafer puts it, "there is no hard-and-fast line between telling and showing" (1983, p. 222). As well, what I tell with my words I often belie by my actions, while my eyes tell a tale all their own. The first is text, as it were; the others, *sub*-text. There is also what I show through my achievements and accomplishments, through my life-*style*, and through the things I own, hairdo I sport, and clothes I wear, which always make some statement about who I am! Even each photograph, each memento on my mantelpiece, communicates a message about what I am like (or want to be *seen* as like), in addition to the story it betokens of a particular past event: the honeymoon in Niagara Falls or the holiday in France.

When *told*, my lifestory on this level reflects the conventions of language and social interaction that are prevalent in the context of my family, culture, or gender as to what is appropriate for both the content and form of a person's self-telling. (See Chapter 4 on "The Larger Stories We Live Within.") The countless possible versions of this level of my lifestory can of course vary very much, both from each other and from the original from which they arise—depending, as we shall see, on my audience, motive, or mood, *and* the medium through which they are expressed. Thus, I can come across one way in a letter, another on the phone, and still another face to face. In general, this level is my *inside-out* story, my public domain, what I select to impart to others, either formally in an autobiography or informally in everyday conversation—or to some side of my own self in the pages of my journal. It is the level of *expression*.

The Outside-In Story

Finally, there is the level of the countless interpretations that others read into part or all of my life (or impose upon it), either informally—in gossip behind my back or feedback to my face—or formally, in a biography, a medical case history, or a psychological "life history" (see Runyan, 1984), a term some researchers use synomously with lifestory. This is the level of *impression*. It is my *outside-in* story, any version of which can be quite inaccurate and incomplete, a mere "storyotype" of who I really am—however influential is my sense of it in shaping my self-concept. To appreciate this influence, we need only remind ourselves of the impact made on us by the impression we *perceived* was held by a parent or employer, lover or friend, even a total stranger.

Such storyotypes are stubbornly strong, as we can discover when encountering some childhood chum, for instance, only to find that their version of us is stuck in the past, resistant to "the facts" of our life in subsequent years—as perhaps ours has been of them! In such situations, we need time to update each other, to negotiate the stories in terms of which we relate to

each other now. Indeed, our ability to keep our impressions of each other
open in this way is one sign of our maturity as persons. (Another is our
reluctance to share with one person our impressions of another before the
two have met, lest the former form a first impression on the strength of a
secondhand story.)

Just as others have outside-in stories of us, then, so we are continually
composing the same of them—likely stories of what their lives are like.
Moreover, driven by a kind of "biographical imperative," we commonly
compose them from the flimsiest of clues—a glance, a gait, a hairdo, an
accent, the length of a hem, the shape of a tie. Indeed, as we shall see in the
next chapter, forming impressions of one another in this superficial manner
is a large part of everyday life, and we can be insatiably curious in going
about it. We need only think of the last time we saw someone shuffling down
the sidewalk in an unusual manner, or overheard a couple arguing at a table
near ours, and said to ourselves: *I wonder what the story is there.* As we
discussed in the last chapter, we can never know completely. Says novelist
E. M. Forster, "we know each other approximately, by external signs, [but]
these serve well enough as a basis for society and even for intimacy"
(Hodgins, 1993, p. 99).

Links and Gaps Between the Levels of Lifestory

Generally, if the outside story is what happens to me, the inside story is
what I *make* of what happens to me and what I tell to myself. In turn, the
inside-out story is what I tell (and show) to others of what I make of what
happens to me, while the outside-in story is what others make of me on their

The Story of My Life

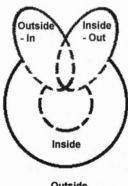

own, with or without my consent. To help us visualize the links between these levels and so put flesh on the accompanying diagram, here are two analogies.

In computer terms, the outside story is the hardware of the system. The inside story, is the software, plus the collection of directories I have assembled with its aid, including whatever file I am into at the moment, part of which fills the screen. The inside-out story is the hard copy I print out for others, who in turn will fashion their own interpretation, outside-in, of what its text might mean.

In publishing terms, my outside story is the physical object of a given novel: the paper, ink, and binding that constitute the thing itself, plus the process by which it was produced. My inside story corresponds to the novel as I *experience* it in the reading: its atmosphere, the unfolding of its plot, its reality within me as an entire story-world. My inside-out story, however, is the summary I make of that world to others—whose versions of it, despite my efforts at "impression management" (Goffman, 1959), each will formulate from nothing more substantial than the notes on the jacket or the design on the front.

Between these levels, of course, are always links and gaps. As for links, the borders that separate them are far from defined. A complex, cyclical relationship exists between them—once again, a hermeneutic circle. In the words of anthropologist Edward Bruner, "experience structures expressions and expressions structure experience" (1986, p. 6). But existence, too, structures experience. The actual *facts* of our life (our facticity) exert at least some influence on our lifestory. External features like a balding head, a physical deformity, or losing a parent in our youth can significantly affect what we *make* of our life on the inside, as can the features of the environment in which we live, as we shall see in the next chapter.

Similarly, impressions structure experience. The way we tell and show ourselves to others generates a picture of what we are like—our abilities and limits. Based on this picture, their treatment of us either opens up certain opportunities or closes them off. Thus, if a team of interviewers is poorly impressed with our handling of their questions, the job will go to another candidate—and our bills will go unpaid. Through a sort of feedback loop, then, the resultant downsizing of our economic existence could lead to sober self-assessment—to a revised version of our lifestory, both inside and, eventually, inside-out.

As for gaps, not only can we never experience the totality of our existence, but neither can we express the totality of our experience, nor can we tell or show *exactly* what we feel or mean. Where telling is concerned, the very language on which we rely forces our words—themselves but arbitrary symbols for actions, relations, and things—into the structures of a particular grammar and syntax. As Spence (1982) has stressed, following the lead of Merleau-Ponty, there are "inevitable slippages between memories of any kind, thoughts, feelings, fantasies, dreams, etc., and a language of intelligible description" (p. 11). Language itself is both vehicle and obstacle, simultaneously helping and inhibiting our communion with ourselves and our communication with others. Says Spence, there is "slippage again between the supposedly shared, perceived, or imputed meaning inferred by the listener" (p. 11). Because of both types of slippage, we encounter the opacity of our stories. Thus, the impressions *others* form of us frequently fail to correspond to—are much less than—what *we* form of ourselves, and for good reason: they cannot experience our experience of ourselves (Laing, 1967).

This failure is easily noticed when we compare the report someone makes on her life in an autobiography (inside-out) with the assessment of that same life by her biographer (outside-in). Indeed, the latter may in many regards be more accurate—as in, truer to "the facts"—than the story she tells of it herself, which often falls prey to delusion concerning the future, fuzzied memory of the past, and distorted perception in the present.

At all levels, then, there is material left over: Our existence forever exceeds our experience, which continually outspans our expression, which is habitually richer than the impression we create in others' eyes. However, we must not think of these levels as therefore quantitative in nature, as if the outside story were simply more than the inside story. Rather, they are qualitatively different, of a different order. Thus the gaps between them are real and must be factored into all of our thinking about human nature and social interaction. Otherwise, we will fail to do justice to the realities of such subtle things as secrecy, self-deception, hypocrisy, even (as we have seen) hypochondria—realities that, however hard to measure, are integral to everyday life.

THE LIBRARY OF OUR LIVES

Novelist Alex Haley once said that "every time an old person dies it's as if a library had burned down" (Polster, 1987, p. 96). Morbid as this statement sounds, it is touchingly true, and we know it, especially if people dear to us have passed away and we have been moved by how much history or lore they have taken with them. But it is true for us all, regardless of our age. As the years roll by, we tuck away an incredible amount of material "in here"—which means, among other things, that "none of us can escape being *interesting*" (p. 3).

Not all of this inner material is especially story-like of course. In the library of our lives are numerous volumes, from cookbooks and phonebooks to works on philosophy and home repair, plus compendia of trivia of countless kinds. Nonetheless, tied to much of this material is, somewhere, an actual event, some concrete touchstone in our personal past. More than a pile of raw figures or brute facts, then, we have a ton of *stories* inside us as well—both *actual* stories and layer on layer of *potential* ones. We ride atop a spinning mass of story *material*, from which we draw each time we express ourselves inside-out: anecdotes and accounts, more or less complete—in some cases only quasi-narrative—of the various experiences we have had and people we have met; of the innumerable things we have suffered and seen, done and endured, thought and felt.

Each element in this material can be combined with others in seemingly endless ways. Furthermore, an element that is in the foreground in one anecdote may be in the background in another. Thus, the same narrative nugget can be told in one context to elicit a laugh—about the time the cow kicked us in the head—while, in another, to sketch the setting for a different tale altogether—about how tough it was growing up on a farm during the Depression. As we saw in the last chapter, it depends on what stimulates our storytelling in the first place, on the mysterious switch that is triggered amid the drift of a given exchange and summons this set of recollections but not that.

On all this material we draw more or less directly all the time—when in conversation (can we imagine everyday chitchat stripped of all storytelling?) or when asked to introduce ourselves or explain who we are. It is always there behind the scenes, ready to be tapped if only the right question is asked, the correct button pressed. It is not that everything we say is packaged in neat story-units, but that this material *en masse* is at the base of all our talk. As we said in Chapter 2, it forms the foundation of our beliefs, our values, our whole mode of being in the world. We also draw on it *in*directly, therefore, when trying to understand something new or to cope with an unfamiliar situation, which simply means that all learning is autobiographical at base (see Brady, 1990). As well, we find allusions to it filling our dreams and traces of it influencing our posture, our gestures, even our organs, insofar as its effects are reflected in the acids in our stomach, the stresses on our heart, and the lines upon our face. We assume it with every breath we breathe and every word we speak—or hear or read. As Sven Birkerts (1994) reminds us, reading itself is a meaningful activity only insofar as, in our encounter with individual words, "we bring our substance to them and make them live." If you will, "the word canisters are empty until we load them from our private reservoirs" (p. 83).

Like stories generally, then, this material is not innocent (Rosen, 1986), not the meaningless meandering of our memory and imagination. On the contrary, it constitutes our sense of self, our very *being,* which is why story is an ontological metaphor. In the words of Roger Schank, "we are the stories we like to tell" (1990, p. 137). Thus, "we tell stories to describe ourselves not only so others can understand who we are but also so we can understand ourselves" (p. 44). Knowing ourselves is inseparable from narrating ourselves. Indeed, "know" and "narrate" may have the same etymological root (Mancusco and Sarbin, 1983; Casey, 1987).

As we suggested last chapter, describing this material as fictional—as malleable, dependent on the context in which it is told—is not to suggest it is a pack of lies, that it has no basis in fact. However, as we shall come to appreciate, an element of fictionalizing is always at work in the process of remembering. Memories are never simply straightforward snapshots of what actually happened, inviolably preserved forever. Whatever else they are, memories are stories. As one author puts it, "we're all storymakers"; making stories is how we make sense of our lives. We continually "story our worlds, our selves, our friends and family" (Gold, 1990, pp. 51, 31). What we want to do now, then, is to catalogue the stories that this storying produces (in the next chapter we consider *how* it produces them), for our inner narrative material is by no means all one piece. But we want to do so not according to their content, which will vary with each person, so much as to their form.

Short Stories Versus Long Stories

To begin, we have short stories and long stories. We have stories that take but a minute to tell—like about what happened at lunch or what we did with our child last evening—and we have stories that can take forever—like the one about our first marriage, our years in the war, or the ups and downs of our career.

Sometimes, stories that could be made quite short and perhaps deserve little air-time get out of hand in the telling. We bring in more detail than we really need and go off on what, to our audience, sound like too many tangents. They would prefer a synopsis instead, not the whole story. As we gauge their growing restlessness, then, we may decide to rein in our tales, abruptly terminating our dissertation with some semi-apology like "but anyway" or "to make a long story short . . . " (In later chapters, we shall return to the role played by the storylistening we receive in the storytelling we do, either encouraging it or cutting it off.)

In contrast, long stories require more air-time since they cover more significant chunks of our life. Where short stories could easily be curtailed, long stories are continually being interrupted, for there is rarely enough time to tell them completely, to do them justice. We can think of long stories as, in turn, being about one of two main topics: sub-plots and chapters.

Subplots Versus Chapters

A *sub*plot is one strand that makes up the *main* plot of a story. (In the next chapter, we explore in more detail the concept of plot in relation to *life*story.) It is woven through it, perhaps runs the full length of it—longitudinally, as it were. It is more or less consequential to the outcome of the main plot, to how it unfolds. For instance, into a movie devoted to the tribulations of its hero trying to solve a crime or defeat an alien may be woven a subplot about the budding romance between two relatively minor characters. This subplot provides a measure of lighter hearted diversion from the unrelenting suspense of the story as a whole. Take it away and even though the story does not fall apart, it is less satisfying to watch, for it is robbed of the periodic suspension of dramatic tension that, for the viewer, keeps the emotional intensity to a manageable level. However, if a story has many such subplots and *all* are removed, the thread of the story will eventually unravel.

But, to make a long story short . . . In our own *life*story are various subplots that we can recount from our memory and imagination. These are the narrative strands that make up our life's unfolding fabric but might not radically undo it if they were absent. (Of course, what seems a subplot today may emerge as the major plot tomorrow, something many of us experience in telling our lifestories over time—in guided autobiography, for instance. See Chapter 5.) We can think of subplots as dimensions of our life over a comparatively long period of time, such as the ups and downs of our involvement with religion, with a certain disability, with a particular parent, or of our lifelong love of baseball or the family farm.

Literary stories and lifestories alike can also be analyzed latitudinally, into specific scenes or chapters. In fact, few notions are as natural as that our lives are divisible into chapters. "If I end this relationship (or quit this job or finish this degree)," it is common to hear, "I'll be ending one chapter and beginning another." While particular subplots may continue to unfold through particular chapters, the latter units have to do with shorter term, more once-and-for-all story chunks—as if they were stories *within* a story. A chapter could be about the summer we replaced the roof at the cottage, the time we hitchhiked to Florida, the year we spent in graduate school, or our brief flirtation with needlepoint or model trains.

Of course, some of the chapters of our life can be long enough and loaded enough to constitute an entire phase or stage of our overall development—biographical development, that is. Compared to these more familiar psychological terms, however, the notion of chapters honors, at once, the storied nature of our lives, their biographical uniqueness (or "novelty"), and the perpetual changes in them over time—yet without the view of change as improvement that stages or phases imply. We would never think of Chapter 12 of a novel as intrinsically better than Chapter 11 or Chapter 1, for each of these others has made its unique contribution to the story as a whole. Instead, it merely *assumes* more because it is farther along on the story line. Thus, each new event it injects or character it introduces is richer in poignancy and meaning because of the greater number of accumulated associations it elicits in us from all we have read so far. The world of the story is not thereby better, only bigger, wider, deeper—or, as we say, "thicker."

Subplots and chapters are integral to the structure of most every long story, like a novel. They make it easier for us to swallow the story by cutting it into chewable segments. Making sense of the stuff of our *life*story is possible in the same way. Otherwise, it might mush too much together in our minds, leaving us confused and overwhelmed—as if lost in our own story. Although the distinction between them can sometimes get blurred, we are usually aware when we are recounting one, when the other, and when we are switching between them: for example, when telling about the summer we replaced the roof on the cottage leads into the much lengthier (indeed, ongoing) story of our relationship with a person we met at the time—who eventually became our spouse! Generally, however, we have some sense that if we are recounting a specific subplot we ought to play down details about any one period in its unfolding and to trace the whole sweep of the relationship or job in question, and so forth. Conversely, if we are into a chapter, then we feel obliged to focus on the particulars of that event or situation, giving it less background and foreground, less preamble and post-amble.

Past Stories Versus Future Stories

A point we can overlook in talking about lifestory is that, like any story, it has a beginning, middle, and end. A story with a beginning but no middle or end would not be much of a story, nor would one with an end but no beginning or middle. In a sense, a story is about the past, present, and future all at once; it is certainly about the future as much as the past. When reading a novel, we are simultaneously looking forward to what lies ahead and backward to what has already happened, continually adjusting our understanding of the latter as the former "unfolds." If we were not involved in this complex process, then the story, *as* a story, would make no sense—no *narrative* sense.

Applying this feature of a literary story to a lifestory, we have not only memories about our past, then, but also fantasies about our future. In fact, the two are often mixed. In many memories, some sense of future is always present, if only a *possible* future that existed in the past. As memory theorist Daniel Schachter puts it, "our stories are built from many ingredients," not only "snippets of what actually happened" but also "thoughts about what *might* have happened" (1996, p. 308).

Certainly, we all have our hopes and dreams, our worries and fears. At the very least, we have our plans, however sketchy their form in our imagination or how poorly we may implement them: plans concerning how our day will proceed, what we will do when we get home, the chat we want to have with our child, or the program we wish to watch on TV. If we were completely plan-*less*, we would be a rather disoriented person. Possessing plans of any kind is one way we manage the potentially paralyzing suspense we could otherwise feel in the face of a future that is always, technically, unknowable.

An example here is decision-making. At root, it is a process of imagining the scenarios to which a given choice could lead—of the direction in which events might unfold if we go with Plan A as opposed to Plan B. It is a process of trying on different stories for size. Although some of us are less future-focused than are others, there is thus no question that if we had no future-sense at all, we would soon be labeled disturbed. We cannot be backward-looking alone. To rearrange a comment made by Danish philosopher Søren Kierkegaard: we may understand life backward, but we have to live it forward.

To appreciate how this is so, we need only listen to ourselves in conversation. Fully half of the stories we relate can concern the future: what we *hope* to accomplish, *fear* might happen, *want* to buy, or *intend* to do—once we win the lottery or find the time. Indeed, from a certain perspective, none of us lives in the *real* world anyway. Rather, we live in a *fantasy* world that we are continually fabricating from the tissues of anticipation through which we gaze—and journey—into time, draped in a cloak of maybes and conjectures, of *what ifs* and *what might bes,* enticed by self-told tales of the unknown (now fearsome, now beguiling) that lies in store ahead of us.

If, as we shall soon consider, our emotions themselves have narrative roots, then it is not just our *re*-flections on the past that stimulate specific feelings within us but also our *pro*-flections on the future. We discussed this in Chapter 2 in terms of how we experience time on the "inside" of our lives, and of the difference between story-time and clock-time. As young people, for example, we are drawn by our future as much as driven by our past, lured by what lies ahead as much as loaded by what has already occurred, pulled by the stories we spin about what we will be when we grow up (or that others spin *for* us) as much as pushed by the tales we have internalized about the way we were. Indeed, it is by our dreams that we grow, that we are drawn forward into our own imagined future, and therefore find our direction—however provisional it may be, as reality repeatedly runs its check on the course of our life. As we mature, do we live any less by such illusion, by wondering or worrying about "what will be"?

Shared Stories

We all have stories that concern us alone—our doings, disappointments, affairs. But we frequently find it difficult to separate our own stories from those involving others. The stories we start telling about ourselves, for example, can quickly turn into stories about the members of our family—our children, partner, parents, even *absent* parents (Schnitzer, 1993)—or about our friends, pets, colleagues, or neighbors: anyone for whom we feel affection, or with whom our fortunes are for better or worse entwined.

One type of shared stories practically all of us carry are *family* stories—funny things that happened to us on vacation, what Daddy did during the war, the time Grandma kept house for us, and so on. Of course, each member of our family will have his or her private anthology—something that can enliven our get-togethers when we compare our respective recollections of our collective past. But whether or not we share the same set of stories, we cannot understand who we are or where we have come from without making *some* reference—sooner or later, explicitly or implicitly—to the set that is ours.

We shall come back to such matters in the next chapter when we look at "The Larger Stories We Live Within." In the meantime, these stories are "rich sources of information about the familial traditions and meaning constructions of the particular people involved" (Parry and Doan, 1994, p. 70). Most of what we know about the lives of our parents or grandparents, for example, is mediated through such stories, though we can rarely nail down their veracity. True or not, they can be understood on two levels: the surface level of what actually happened—of who did what and when—and the level beneath the surface, where important messages are often conveyed, and myths proclaimed, about "the way things are" in the family and the world. As Elizabeth Stone writes, family stories "are usually teaching stories" that "make known its norms and mores" and "underscore . . . the essentials, like unspoken and unadmitted family policy on marriage or illness. . . . Or who the family saints and sinners are, or how much anger can be expressed and by whom" (1988, p. 7). The importance of family stories, especially if left unexamined, will become even clearer in Chapter 5 as we see how they "reveal the major sources of authorship that were influential in penning the scripts" of our lives—authorship we need to critique if we are ever to author ourselves (Parry and Doan, 1994, p. 70f).

Specific Stories Versus General Stories

On the one hand, we have stories of specific things we have witnessed or experienced or done; things that stand out as unusual or unique; that stick stubbornly in our mind's eye, year after year; that we just can't forget. On the other hand, we have stories that are general in nature: not about individual incidents etched indelibly within us, but about "the kind of thing I *used* to do"—the countless times we went tobogganing behind the house, or shopping with Grannie, or the dozen of trips to the doctor about this ailment or that.

Among such numberless occasions, we may have no recollection of any *in particular*, though we have no doubt that all of them took place, and indeed we can still recall the feel of typical scenes. But our memories of these occasions have somehow merged into one extended memory, just as the lights of passing cars blend into one long stream of light in a time-lapse photograph of a freeway at night. The stories we have of specifics are what memory theorists call episodic memories. More general ones are "*re*episo-dic," for though based on a series of real episodes, each technically unique, the series is so long and the episodes so many that they have become the norm, not separate and distinct (Neisser, 1986).

Fuzzy Stories Versus Focused Stories

We have stories that can be hazy and unfocused, like those related to our earliest memories. That is, we may have a vague recollection of doing such and such when we were little but find it difficult to summon any anecdotes to substantiate it. At the same time, we have other stories that are pointed and precise, whose details continue to be clear to us despite the intervening years—like those about certain crises we have long-since undergone but that seem to represent major turning points in our life-path.

Related to this distinction is that of partial versus complete, or loose-ended versus resolved. On the one hand, we have bits of stories that rumble around inside us, the beginnings of stories, as it were—a few scraps of mental images, and so forth—but nothing that adds up to a particular tale, nothing terribly tellable, though in time it may work its way into some other tale instead. On the other hand, we have complete story units, each with a definite beginning, middle, and end—even its own moral or "point," whether or not we ever spell it out (Linde, 1993; Polster, 1987).

Ordinary Stories Versus Extraordinary Stories

We tend to tell stories about what stands out as unique. Imagine telling a neighbor in excruciating detail about washing the dishes, something you do every day. No matter how glamorous you made it sound, you would soon get the message that you were boring your audience, if not by your delivery then by your detail. Events worth narrating are those that depart from the norm. Unless ordinary events can be turned into *extra*ordinary ones (and here some hyperbole can help!)—unless they can be transformed into adventures—they are better left untold.

What makes an adventure is the novelty of the event at its core, the unusualness of its occurrence. What is reportable (Linde, 1993) in everyday conversation is what goes beyond the everyday. Whenever we congregate with our companions to swap stories, we thus tacitly agree to trade tales that go beyond raw regurgitation of what everyone already knows—as in, one event tacked tediously to another in the breathless and-then-and-then fashion we quickly tire of when our ten-year-old insists on recounting the movie he or she saw the night before.

Signature Stories

Certain stories, we *like* to tell. These are the tales about ourselves that we trot out at parties when meeting someone new, or in those Hello-my-name-is situations at a workshop or conference, or when trying to create a particular impression in others' eyes. Tried and true, practiced and polished, they often take the form of "I'll never forget the time" stories—stories about the time our dog died, or we met our mate, or we told off old so-and-so once and for all.

These stories stand out like mountain peaks above our memory's broad, mostly cloud-covered plain. If we were ever to write a formal autobiography, it is around such stories we might well construct our narrative. We can think of them as *signature* stories, for they are accounts of ourselves that are relatively safe to tell, anecdotes with which we are willing to go public. They are stories that make a statement of sorts, that communicate things about us we do not mind people knowing, perhaps even *want* them to know. This is why, despite us, they can come gushing from our mouths to people we have barely met, yet with whom, for whatever reason, we choose to "open up" (Pennebaker, 1990).

Just one of our signature stories, however, can reveal a great deal about us if we lay it out and study it like we might a piece of literary text. (In Chapter 5, in fact, we suggest that this is exactly what we do, not just to evaluate its content and meaning but also to pry ourselves loose from the particular interpretation it places on pivotal life events, thus preparing the way for us to restory our life as a whole.) It can reveal much about the ways we compose our lives in our memory and imagination (or would like to be perceived by others), and the ways of characterizing ourselves and emplotting our lives to which we are typically inclined. (See *Bill's Iron Lung Story*, following page.) If you will, signature stories are like parables that give those with eyes to see a glimpse of our "storying style," something we shall say more about in the following chapter. Whether happy or sad, about good times or bad, they say something about what turns us on or makes us tick; about the turning points in our path; about why our life has taken the course it has. As such, they are often "origin stories" that say, basically, *and that's why I am the way I am—and am* not (Bruner, 1990).

Our signature stories also indicate something about our fundamental beliefs, our convictions and values, habits and idiosyncracies; something about our hopes and fears, and our limits—about how far we can be pushed or how far we will go. We may be keen to tell them, therefore, because, whether we realize it or not, they undergird the personal "myth" which (unconsciously) guides our life (see Keen, 1993; Pearson, 1989; Feinstein et al, 1988; Campbell and Moyers, 1988). For this reason, our signature stories can have a legendizing impulse running through them, especially the more frequently we tell them or the more positively they are heard. (Thus, the fish that got away grows longer with each telling, or the love we lost more lovely, and so on.) Indeed, Freud compared the stories we have of our childhood "to the legends and traditions of a nation's prehistory, because both have been gathered and interpreted to fit later ideas" (Charmé, 1984, p. 42). Such stories can often screen from present awareness darker, more serious matters about our past (Spence, 1982).

As central as signature stories are, however, we are not psychoanalysts ourselves. Thus, apart from our observations here about what such stories are and why they "work," we offer no grand theory as to how they are formed in the first place, or why they get formed around these sets of events and not those. Like much about composing a life, this may remain largely a mystery.

BILL'S IRON LUNG STORY

When I was two years old, I contracted polio—as did my two sisters. Three of countless casualties in an epidemic that hit our region in the early 1950s, we enjoyed the benefit neither of Medicare nor of the Salk vaccine that has supposedly now eradicated the virus from the globe. One sister nearly died, from paralysis of the trachea; the other was left severely and permanently disabled. As for me, the disease attacked my diaphragm, the muscle system just below the lungs that, bellows-like, makes it possible to breathe.

For two weeks, early in my illness, I was consigned to an iron lung—a Catscan-sized, tank-shaped apparatus timed to assist respiration from the outside rather than the inside, as does the modern respirator. Without it, I would have died, unable to catch my breath. With it, I survived to tell the tale. In that tale, I am in a cold, grey room specially reserved for such equipment. No one else is around. It is not a room gaily papered with teddybears and smiley faces like a children's ward today, but drab and barren, for my ordeal unfolded in an era when hospitals were less for getting well than for being sick. Outside the two barred windows of my solitary cell is the ghostly, midwinter fog of the port city where we lived at the time.

Dismal as it sounds, I have always liked this story. Indeed, on dozens of occasions I've heard myself recount it, often at social events or parties, when conversations sometimes turn to life-threatening diseases we've all suffered but survived—occasions when a little sympathy never hurts to get your way, or at least some attention over the hors d'oeuvres. I've always enjoyed how this story portrays me, the light in which it shows me: a tiny child-hero, hemmed-in and powerless, with no choice but to lie there and take it—alone.

The problem is, the story isn't true—at least, the bit about the iron lung. As it turns out, I'd had it all wrong. According to my parents, whose recollections I finally solicited forty years after what I'd figured was the fact, it never took place. Oh sure, they were worried about their little darling and lovingly ensured I didn't go outside to play following my diagnosis. And, true, they refused to treat it lightly when later that season I contracted pneumonia, which meant that for a few days I was placed in an oxygen tent and had my tummy lathered with the 1950s equivalent of Vicks Vapo-Rub. But that was apparently it. Nothing more dramatic or traumatic occurred. I'd trumped it up, they politely implied.

With equal politeness, I implied they'd done the same with *their* version, that being my parents didn't automatically place them nearer the truth. Indeed, the truth, I ventured, had had to be doctored because too difficult to admit—that they had been powerless to care for me; that in my toughest hour they'd abandoned me to a machine. Naturally, till we find whatever records may have been kept at the time, we'll never know whose memory—if either's—is right.

Yet, right or not, this story has continued to mean something to me, even after my parents' "correction." Why?, I ask myself. What's been in it for me? Why have I kept it in my repertoire—or *composed* it, as the case may be? Did I not secretly suspect it all these years? What is it *about*? What personal myth has it tacitly confirmed? What aspect of my character, my relationships, my ongoing life in the world might I have invented it to undergird? What failures, physical or other, has it allowed me to excuse? For what sibling oneupmanship has it supplied me with support? To what deep patterns of thinking and feeling has it given subtle sanction?

Secret Stories

In contrast to signature stories are secret ones. Secrets are stories—partial or complete, fuzzy or precise, innocent or dark (skeletons in the closet, for instance)—that we tend to keep to ourselves. That is, unless we encounter some trustable soul on whom we can unload them. In other words, we would probably like to tell them someday—provided the right audience. Fueled by what can be called "the autobiographical imperative" (Randall, 1995)— by the need to be known, to tell our story straight—our secrets, too, want eventually to "out." The right audience could be a close friend, a therapist, or the proverbial stranger-on-the-train we expect never to meet again. It matters not who, as long as we feel that, with him or her, the story will be safe. Until we have this feeling, however, the cost of maintaining our silence may force us to lead a secret life. This was the case with gay author Paul Monette (1992). To the autobiographical chronicle of his long, slow journey to come out of the closet, Monette assigns a subtitle whose poignancy tells all: *Half a Life Story*.

Public Versus Private, Surface Versus Deep

Related to the signature-secret distinction is that of public versus private. The former are stories we dare to relate only when on our guard—for example, in a professional setting—or when out and about. They are relayed using the smiles, the demeanor, the conventions of social intercourse prevalent in the circles in which we move. But we tell them from our persona, not our core. By contrast, the latter are accounts of ourselves that we allow to come out when at home or with people we trust, with whom we are comfortable enough to "let down our hair."

Related to the public-private distinction is that between surface and deep—or, if you will, cover versus covered, or presenting versus real. Surface stories are relatively easy to tell, close to the tip of our consciousness. Deep stories are more elusive—even to ourselves. They are the stories behind the stories, stories too painful, embarrassing, or complex to tell. For example, on the surface we may prattle on uproariously to our fellow partyers about the time we got locked in the bathroom and had to climb through the window in the middle of winter—dressed only in our pajamas. Meanwhile, the real story is that our alcoholic father had deliberately shut us in, as punishment for protesting against another of the rages that made a nightmare of our youth.

"Deep story" has an additional meaning, however. It is the story that, until we have outgrown it, cannot be articulated, even to ourselves. It is too deep for words. Yet it profoundly informs how we think and feel. It is our guiding myth—not in the sense of something untrue, but *so* true, so bound up with how we see ourselves in the world, so nonnegotiable, therefore, that we accept it as the way things are. It is not something we can see (or tell), but something we see (or tell) *through*; thus, part of our facticity.

Untold Stories

No matter how many stories we *could* tell, to others or just ourselves (as in secrets), there are countless more we leave untold altogether. These make up the material "between the lines' —or the *sub*text—of our life. While hints of this material regularly swarm our dream-world, some can be, for all practical purposes, inaccessible, so deep as to be unknown. Commenting on the tendency of readers to *under*read a novel, critic Frank Kermode writes of the "narrative secrets" that any story of substance will withhold from us under even our most rigorous reading (1980). The stories we leave untold *to ourselves*, if you will, are the narrative secrets that lie just beyond the edge of even the most scrupulous *self*-reading.

As any psychoanalyst will confess, the very concept of untold stories is enticing. It piques our curiosity; it arouses what C. S. Lewis has called our "narrative lust" (1966, p. 103), our desire to know the unknown. In terms of the levels of lifestory we looked at earlier, however, it conveys two ideas. The first is that not all of our experience can be expressed to others. That is, not all of our inside story can be transferred to the level of inside-out. There can be several reasons for this.

One is the demands of diplomacy or discretion. That is, we want to avoid hurting others' feelings or shattering their illusions, and so we decide that certain matters are better left unsaid. Another is because of deliberate deception—if not by outright lying then by cloaking what we say in hints and half-truths in order to mislead our listener. Another reason is simple forgetfulness, a phenomenon we shall touch on in the next chapter. Still another is not merely shyness but an inordinate need for privacy, even for what one writer has called "erasing personal history" to avoid the "encumbering thoughts" of others and so set ourselves free to be whomever we wish (Castenada, 1975).

As well, we may not express all of our experience because of a certain impression we want another person to form of us. We want them to see us as unavailable, aloof; we want to hide from them how deeply we care, lest they be frightened of our intentions and pull away. Or we want to retain an air of mystery to entice them to take more interest, ask us about our past, and pursue the clues we cannily toss them about the exotic places we have visited or people we know. Or it may be because of a limited vocabulary, meaning we simply can't find the words with which to relate what we have experienced—or perhaps are in the process of experiencing, because events are still unfolding and thus have not yet reached the sort of resolution that would render them tellable. (In this case, they remain unfinished stories.) As we shall see in the next chapter, we can also leave our inside story untold on the level of inside-out because of our need to edit. That is, we routinely do not tell others everything going on in our lives, and neither do we tell ourselves. Instead, we screen out vast portions of our existence—our emotions, thoughts, memories, daydreams—seconds (or less) after experiencing them.

To refer to the stories we leave untold is also to say that not all of our existence gets experienced in the first place. As it were, nine-tenths of the iceberg lies beneath the surface. As we shall see in the next chapter, the plotting in which we inevitably engage leads us, automatically, to *ex*clude from our consciousness and attention, our memory and imagination, far more than we *in*clude. As Erving Polster sees it, "the raw material for stories is always being formed. Each moment in a person's life hosts an endless number of events. Considering the abundance of this treasure, relatively few stories emerge" (1987, p. 21).

Much of the material that gets left unstoried on both borders—between existence and experience and between experience and expression—may not be utterly lost, however. As we shall see in Chapter 5, it constitutes a kind of compost heap—what one writer calls "the detritus of my history" (Truitt,

1987, p. 209)—from which a fuller version of ourselves, a more livable lifestory, may later spring.

ONE EVENT YET MANY VERSIONS

What makes everyday life endlessly fascinating (and frustrating) is how two people can go through the same event yet spin from it two different versions. As we considered in Chapter 2, this keeps the question of truth, and of true stories, constantly alive—not to mention what is "an event" in the first place, a philosophical question we are not prepared to wrestle with here. But it is not just that one person picks up on some details of what happened while the second notices others. Each person seems to experience it in fundamentally distinctive ways, to make sense of it on significantly different levels.

Such differences stand out clearly when we compare how our local newspaper reports a particular world event with the coverage given it by a national newspaper—or a foreign journal, or a cheap tabloid, or a highbrow magazine a month after the fact. Furthermore, the same figures we fancy could never lie can be made to support many different facts, and from one set of statistics "spin doctors" can extract a broad set of stories. Closer to home, a tidbit about our neighbour can get twisted out of all recognition as it makes its way from mouth to ear down the length of Gossip Row.

Variations on the versions of a given event are easy to see and laugh at when they concern the lives of others. However, when they concern events in ours, we can be blissfully unaware of the range of ways we represent them to ourselves. A number of factors contribute to this width.

For one, the way we relate a given experience varies with our audience. As we have said, stories and storytelling are purpose-driven, context-driven, and "we"-driven. We tell *about* something *to* someone, and we want that someone to receive (and believe) what we are giving and to return a particular response—be it sympathy, reinforcement, or advice. Thus, what we tell a dear friend about our divorce may be significantly different—more elaborate, with more of "the gory details"—than the version we share with our mother, our lover, our lawyer, or our boss. Events in themselves never speak for themselves but, as Polster says, are merely raw material, notoriously vulnerable to revision according to whatever effect we want our tale of them to have.

Related to audience is motive. Prancing about with a lampshade on our head at the St. Patrick's Day party will likely take a different narrative form when we recount it to our fellow Irishmen than when we confess our sins to the parish priest, or check in with others at AA, or talk out our troubles with a therapist. The motives behind telling any of our stories are many and often mixed, whether to entertain, show support, instill guilt, arouse suspicion, or accomplish several purposes at once. Related to motive is context. Different social settings elicit some of our stories and inhibit others. We tend not to tell the same tidbits about ourselves at a religious gathering as we would in the locker room, the boardroom, the powder room, or the courtroom, and the joust of stories for which it is routinely the arena.

Related to all these factors is our sheer distance in time from the events our stories concern. Things change in our memory with the passing of years—in importance, in meaning, in perceived impact on the course of our life. Thus, today's horrific accident, too terrible for words, commonly turns into tomorrow's tragedy, and with the passing weeks, is reduced even further in dramatic significance. Like yesterday's news, it gets *de*-genre-ated—poetically downgraded from major tragedy this week to minor one the next, and from high adventure the following month to comic *mis*adventure the month after that. Indeed, from the vantage point of sufficient decades it may be entirely transformed, from, say, a disaster in the beginning to a farce in the end, or else into a sanitized parable of the vicissitudes of a long, full life.

Such de- or re-genre-ation is an example of the empowering potential of the lifestory metaphor, of how it opens the door to an optimistic view of our development as persons (a point we return to in Chapters 5 and 7) by supporting the old saw about time—or story-time—healing all wounds. It is also an example of how our memories of past events—events we may believe have happened "just so"—are ever only *versions*. If we could go back and re-live those events we might notice different things and so form different versions. Though the real past is fixed, then, the remembered past is not. As Sartre scholar Stuart Charmé, puts it: "While it is true on one level that a person has but one life and one past, it is not so obvious that there is only one authoritative story of his or her life. There can be different 'versions' of the story of one's life, each presenting a different text for interpretation" (1984, p. 52).

THE NOVELTY OF OUR LIVES

All of this talk about the different versions we can spin from a given event, the various levels of lifestory, and the many types of story material, told and untold, that lie layered inside us, could leave us with the impression that our personalities are split—if not in a psychological sense, then in a poetic one. It could lead us to believe that our personal identity is, story-

wise, an anthology at best, a narrative collage that is intrinsically disconnected. However, most of us feel instinctively that the opposite is true; that
our many stories with their many versions ultimately converge; that they
stem from and refer to a single, central story line, however winding it
be—"the story of my life" as a whole.

One way to understand how our many stories can nonetheless be one is
to recall how a full-length novel is never the single story it appears. Though
it may possess a central story line, it has no center as such. It always has
many stories spinning about within it. Indeed, there are as many stories in
a given novel as there are points of view from which to view it. For instance,
there is the story contained in each chapter or conveyed by each subplot.
There is the story the author had in mind for it to turn into before, during,
and after composing it. There is the story as mediated by the narrator
through whom it is told. There is the story that each of its characters would
perceive it to be from one chapter to the next, if they were inclined to talk
about it. Finally, there is the story it is seen to be by everyone who reads
it—who, in turn, as they talk about it with other readers, will entertain a
succession of theories as to what sort of story it is. Yet, despite these many
stories, actual or potential, a novel is still only one, the one within which,
between the covers, the many are contained.

With such insights before us, we can extend the metaphor of life-as-story
to that of life-as-novel—the novelty of our lives. As the French writer
Gustave Flaubert once said, "everyone's life is worth a novel." The notion
of novelty brings together the storied aspects of our lives with our uniqueness. "Every person born into this world," says philosopher Martin Buber,
"represents something new, something that never existed before, something
original and unique" (Moustakas, 1967, p. 27). The story material that
comprises our soul is unique to us. No one's library is quite like ours.
Though this can be the source of loneliness, that is, because no one therefore
ever *really* knows us, it can be the source of healthy pride as well—the
realization how special (as in, our own *species*) each one of us is. Just as
every novel creates *and is* a universe all its own, so each of us, as a *living*
novel, tends to live in our own little world.

The notion of the novelty of our lives also highlights the dynamic
integrity of our lifestory material over time. Like *any* story, it "goes
somewhere," with its own momentum and direction. It also underlines the
essential continuity of that material. That is, we change continually, and the
memories and imaginations (fantasies, hopes, illusions) that we entertain
about our lives today can be quite different from those of ten years ago, or
even yesterday. However, the sense that all of these memories and imagin-

ings, despite their many permutations over time, are ultimately and uniquely *ours*—this is rock bottom. It constitutes what philosopher Anthony Paul Kerby (1991) calls "the prenarrative level of experience" or the "quasi-narrative background structure of our lives." Such a background, he writes, "accounts for the ongoing sense of orientation and purpose our lives generally exhibit" and is "the condition of possibility for the stories we tell of ourselves" (p. 7f). As we are saying here, lifestories are lived before they are told.

When we say dynamic integrity, then, we are referring not just to the directionality of our lifestory but also to a fundamental drive to integrate inside ourselves all our understandings of all our doings. Despite the fact, as we considered in Chapter 2, that many pieces of our lifestory run parallel within us, this is the drive to do what the novelist does, which is to continually pull a myriad events and emotions, details and developments, relationships and possibilities into an ever wider story-world that has a coherence and followability (Kerby, 1991) all its own. In this respect, our lifestory—like any story—is always greater than the sum of its components, just as "we" are always more than the parts of our body. Thus, what the novelist does consciously in her art—create narrative order out of what is otherwise chaos—each of us does constantly, if *un*consciously, in our life. Conceived as a kind of "autobiographical imperative" (Randall, 1995), this drive is linked to what Sartre terms the "fundamental project" that we must each undertake to weave the stuff of our life into a meaningful narrative that, psychologically, affords us a home and an anchor amid the immensities of time and space. The result of such weaving, says Sartre, is our own "true novel" (Charmé, 1984).

EMOTIONS AND STORIES

As we said in Chapter 2, stories undergird not only our identity but also our emotions. Of course, modern medical science has considerably demystified the emotional dimension of human life by showing how much of it has physiological roots. In other words, we feel the way we feel in certain situations or with certain people, or our moods swing this way and that, largely because of straightforward factors like our blood sugar level, the amount of sleep we are getting, or an imbalance in our body chemistry due to heredity or diet—an imbalance which medication might easily right. Indeed, for extreme advocates of the medical model, our psychical states— our emotions, our thoughts, and especially our dreams—have little substance in their own right, except as epiphenomema of our physiological condition. But our emotions, we believe, have narrative roots as well. Indeed, what we call our temperament or disposition is in several respects a byproduct of our involvement in stories: not just those we read or hear about others (fictional or not) but, more to the point, those we tell ourselves (and/or internalize from others) *about ourselves*. This point deserves some defense.

The events of our lives are neutral in themselves—neither positive nor negative—until we interpret them as such within the context of what we perceive as the movement of our life as a whole. "There is nothing either good or bad," says Shakespeare, "but thinking makes it so." A given emotional response to a given situation is thus partially a function of the lifestory into which we see that situation fitting. Emotion, says one philosopher, "is the acceptance of, the assent to live according to, a certain sort of story" (Nussbaum, 1989, p. 218). Put another way, our emotions are our (aesthetic) reactions to the stories we tell ourselves about what is going on. These stories construct the meaning and value of the events of our lives. As Zen master John Daido Loori puts it, "anger is only a thought. It is nothing more than the mind getting away from the present moment. Anger usually has to do with what has already happened, or what is going to happen next" (1993, p. 202). When the lifestory we entertain of ourselves changes, therefore, our emotions change as well. Since this is a provocative notion— that our feelings are byproducts of our lifestories and change accordingly— we need to consider it more closely.

The best example is in relation to movies and novels. Who would deny that such stories elicit our emotions? We need only recall our embarrassment at getting caught crying during a critical point in a film. Moreover, we often choose certain films to take us out of one mood and put us in another. But why do they have this power? Movies are not real life—we all know that—and novels are technically just words on a page. True, yet in reading those words we get mysteriously enmeshed in a narrative process that *moves* us through time (hence e-*motion*), from a beginning to an end—a process that acts on some curious mix of memory and imagination and, out of thin air, stimulates an entire sequence of feelings, from suspense to surprise and from sadness to satisfaction. Indeed, a whole cluster of feelings can hang with us for days, as we wander through our lives still under the story's spell.

Stories we hear about others can move us too, often by triggering stories about ourselves. An anecdote from a friend updating us on a former lover—someone we have not thought about for years—can unleash a flood of reminiscence about bygone days. In turn, these reminiscences can generate a swirl of sweetness and sadness, of regret or relief for what might have been, for what we know now but were ignorant of at the time. More to the point, the story material *of our own life* can move us. In fact, the resonance of this material with the stories in movies and novels is what gives depth to our emotional responses to them in the first place (Beach, 1990), whether or not we are conscious of such resonance or of what, within our *life*story, might be its source. This leads to two insights.

The first, which we return to in Chapter 5, is regularly expounded by literary critics who insist that it is through our exposure to great fiction that our emotions (and imagination) are most truly educated, are shaped and refined, stretched and enriched (see Frye, 1963; Booth, 1988; Birkerts, 1994). The second is closer to home. It is that the fictions of many (though maybe not all) of our own memories—and fantasies—stimulate emotions inside us, and frequently according to familiar genres.

At the base of our depressed state, if you will, is a tragic tale. The despair we feel in the face of a particular event is tied to a story that says, essentially, "this is another setback, like all the others, a sure sign that my life is going nowhere, that I'll die penniless and alone." Hope, on the other hand, is tied to a tale of the romantic or adventure genre: "yes, I've had my troubles, and I'll have more to come, but I always come through them a better person. Everything will turn out in the end. Besides, it's always darkest just before the dawn."

Of course, we can flip from one version to another, from seeing the glass of our life as half empty to seeing it half full. Indeed, in a matter of minutes a wide range of spirits can rise and fall within us, and we can go through a lifetime of emotions—our inner world is that complex, that subtle. Yet no one, no matter how close to us, may clue to the swing of our moods if they fail to notice the moistness in our eyes or the smile that lingers on our lips. Moreover, what triggers such swings can be the simplest, most delicate occurrences: a news flash, a chance meeting, a twinge of pain, the receipt of a letter, the sound of an old tune, the whiff of a familiar perfume. Depending how "moody" we are, or how easily swayed from our daily tasks, we may secretly seek to limit the fluctuations such stimuli prompt, either by sticking to routine or by withdrawing from the (always unpredictable) flow of ordinary life.

We could continue in this vein: How much of the emotion of love is tied to a dream about the future—in our rocking chairs, together on the porch— and to a remembrance of things past—the magic of our first meeting, the sweetness of reconciliation after our first fight? And what about nostalgia and hate? The point is, we do not feel in a vacuum. If we are sad, we are probably sad *about* something, and identifying that something involves telling a story. Our emotions are tied to story-lines. Trigger different story-lines for plotting particular situations and different emotions arise. This insight has powerful implications that we shall return to later, especially as we consider the consequences of *re*storying. A very important one concerns the connection between the development of our emotional life *as we age*—for example, the deepening or nuancing of our reactions to even the most ordinary events—and the everchanging vastness, the sedimental layeredness, of our inner story world (see Casey, 1987).

Another implication is that the story-lines of our lives do not get laid down inside us in a vacuum either. As we shall see in the next chapter when we consider the narrative environments by which we are shaped, we learn these story-lines—*we learn our emotions*— "in the same way that we learn our beliefs—from our society. . . . They are taught, above all, through stories" (Nussbaum, 1989, p. 217). For instance, if we have grown up in a neighborhood where we have known only poverty and violence, and where the tales we have heard and witnessed have mainly been tales of woe, then we could easily conclude that our individual existence has little meaning or merit, and our prospects for the future meager at best. Long after we have moved away, we may find it hard to hope.

CONCLUSION

Becoming aware of the countless stories of our lives—the many kinds and levels—is crucial to understanding how we have come to compose ourselves in the ways we have. And it is fundamental to distancing ourselves sufficiently from how we are habitually immersed in the details of our lives so that we can decide how we might want to *change* our lives, which is our subject in Chapter 5. But before we explore the process of "storying" our lives, let us be reminded of the poetic complexity we each possess.

We are all different, or, as we are suggesting here, "novel." But it is not just that we live in different bodies and do different things. Rather, we live in different story-worlds. That is, we are at different points along the plot lines of different *life*stories. In turn, these are comprised of different story material that we can re-version in virtually unlimited ways and, as we shall see in the next chapter, can relate to from various angles in varying proportions in a variety of contexts. Furthermore, this material, which can elicit in us such a wide range of emotional responses, has roots in a particular configuration of larger stories still, within which we make sense of our world. The storied complexity of even the simplest life thus makes each of us unfailingly interesting. Says neuropsychologist, Oliver Sacks: "Biologically, physiologically, we are not so different from each other; historically, as narratives—we are each of us unique" (1985, p. 111).

Chapter 4

The Storying of Our Lives

Because we are engaged in a day-by-day process of self-invention . . . both the
past and the future are raw material, shaped and reshaped by each individual.
Mary Catharine Bateson (1989)

INTRODUCTION

We now have an appreciation of how many and varied are the stories of our
lives, and thus how complicated a lifestory can be. But realizing the richness
of our story material is only the first step in the restorying process. The
second is considering where it has come from and why it possesses the form
and content it does. In other words, the narratives by which we identify ourselves
and move through the world are by no means cast in stone. On some level,
we make them up. The purpose of this chapter is to look at how we do this.

In pursuit of this purpose, three concepts need introduction since they
are the backdrop to what follows: *Composing a Life*, *Life as Text*, and
Storying Style. After these, we consider in detail two important matters:
first, *What a Story Is*—where we apply the concepts of plot, character, genre,
and point of view to both literary story and lifestory; second, *The Larger
Stories We Live Within*—where we examine the social systems that shape
us, in terms of their poetic structure, their narrative environment, and the
kind of coauthoring that occurs within them.

COMPOSING A LIFE

In an important book tracing the lives of herself and four of her female
friends, anthropologist Mary Catharine Bateson (1989) offers a rich meta-

phor for the process by which we make ourselves up. It is "composing a life." With this as her title, she expounds a vision of each person's life as a work of "*improvisatory* art," for it involves the combination of "familiar and unfamiliar components in response to new situations, following an underlying grammar and an evolving aesthetic" (p. 3). More recently, Bateson (1993) has extended her metaphor beyond its obvious connection with art and music (we speak of composing a song) to "the stories you make about your life, and the stories you tell first yourself and then to other people, the stories you use as a lens for interpreting experience as it comes along" (p. 41).

"Composing a life" relates well, we feel, to Sartre's "fundamental project": the peculiar work-in-progress that is "the cumulative structure of meaning that unfolds slowly in the course of a life and links together a person's past, present, and future into a coherent whole" (Charmé, 1984, p. 50). Sartre's belief that this project has "literary qualities" (p. 84) is reinforced by Bateson's idea of using our lifestories as a lens for interpreting experience. In turn, this idea supports the insight that, as one critic puts it, "stories are not innocent" (Rosen, 1986, p. 236). Even the sweetest bedtime story is laden with values, loaded with biases, bent on mediating a *moral* and pushing a point.

The same is true for the stories we entertain about ourselves. As Sartre stresses in the epigraph at the beginning of Chapter 3, we see everything that happens to us *through* them. They are not mere still lifes benignly lining the halls of our memory, but windows through which we gaze upon our world. What we see is what their size and shape—and opacity—*allow* us to see. In this respect, "we *become* the autobiographical narratives by which we 'tell about' our lives" (Bruner, 1987, p. 15). Our stories are not neutral; they are linked to both our identity and our ideology. The focus of this chapter, then, is this loaded, *literary* process whereby we fashion both our life and our world.

LIFE AS TEXT

Bruner makes the provocative statement that "there is no such thing psychologically or subjectively as 'life itself' " (1987, p. 13). What each of us calls "my life" is ultimately our own creation. It is not a given entity but something we compose, as we might a novel or poem. A metaphor that supports this vision, simultaneously underlying the story metaphor and honoring the languaged nature (or *poeisis*) of human being, is that of "life as text" (see McAdams, 1994; White and Epston, 1990). Insists Bruner, with colleague Susan Weisser, " 'lives' are texts: texts that are subject to revision, exegesis, reinterpretation, and so on" (1991, p. 129). Indeed, "it is only by textualization that one can 'know' one's life" (p. 136). Moreover, it is only by textualization that one can know the life of someone else. As we shall see in considering character, all we ever have of another person (as they of us) is an "imaginal entity" (Moore, 1992), an interpretation we formulate from (the texts of) their words and actions, gestures and appearances.

This leads to the corresponding notion that our life has tex*ture,* in at least two senses. First, as Sartre saw, its structure "resembles a literary text" (Charmé, 1984, p. 52) in terms of its richness and depth, and the layers of meaning that can be extracted from it. Second, to borrow a term from singer Carole King, it is a "tapestry" of intertwining traces from the texts both of others' lives and of the many larger stories in which we are enmeshed. All such texts comprise the *con*text of our life—though how profoundly they "saturate" and "construct" our lifestories is a matter of debate (see Gergen, 1991; Shotter and Gergen, 1989). Those involved in the debate refer to this intertwining as intertextuality, the state in which "every text is related to every other text" (Rosenau, 1992, p. 36).

With language as our loom, then, every one of us is a weaver, continually fashioning and refashioning the fabric of our being from the countless events and influences, circumstances and relationships, that are its content on a day-to-day basis. We are forever turning our existence (outside story) into text (inside story), and subsequently into the public texts of the words and actions through which we express ourselves to others (inside-out story).

STORYING STYLE

As we saw in the last chapter, there is more than one way to story an event. Recounting a minor accident in which we were involved while driving home, one of us tells a tale tinged with tragedy. Our tone, expressions, gestures—all support a tragic rendition. The other casts our account in a different genre. Instead of a tale of woe, it is a comedy of errors, a hilarious adventure, the stuff of a good laugh. Of course, one of us may simply have been having a bad day, and so saw everything in it (including the accident) through grey-colored glasses. But it may also be a difference in disposition at work, in temperament, which can be partly but never completely explained in terms of our biochemical makeup or genetic heritage.

Literary connoisseurs are keenly aware of such differences. Presented with an anonymous piece of prose they are adept at identifying it as the work of one author but not another. "That's from Hemingway, I bet," they may say, "not from Steinbeck. It's just not Steinbeck's *style*." Though the concept of style is far from clearcut, we can think of it as that unsayable something, that one quality above everything else, that separates the work of one writer—or musician or artist—from another. Yet, a consideration of style is central to the analysis not only of literary stories but of lived ones as well, of the stories we *are*.

Everyone of us has our particular "ways." Though others can usually pick them out better than we can ourselves, we each have our little mannerisms, our typical phrases and sayings, our particular rituals and routines, our trademark habits of wearing our hair or waving our hands. Furthermore, whether we imitate or inherit it, we each possess a telltale tone of voice, a peculiar posture, a "presence" that sets us apart. Commonly, these become more pronounced (or set) as our lives wear on. As the saying goes, "the older we grow, the more like ourselves we become." Our thesis here, however, is that much of what constitutes our personal style is rooted in a particular mode of storying the events and people that make up our lives. Our life*style* is linked to our life*story*. As advocates of narrative therapy are fond of saying: "the story lives us" (White, 1995, p. 15).

The concept of storying style is not without precedent. Modern psychology has helped us accept, for instance, that people have different personality types and unique learning styles, distinctions that concern the peculiar ways we take in the world, relate to others, process our emotions, and so forth. While the notion of *storying* styles is not intended to displace these other distinctions, it suggests that people are different in the same vast range of ways that a novel by Hardy is different from one by Updike or Oates. By focusing on the unique manner in which we make sense of our lives in storied form, it seriously honors the novelty of our lives.

WHAT A STORY IS

The notion of storying style confronts us with what seems the simplest question: *What is a story?* Unfortunately, it is as difficult to answer as it is easy to ask. "Through long practice I know how to tell a story," confesses author Ursula Le Guin, "but I'm not sure I know what a story is" (1989, p. 37). Echoes philosopher Hayden White, story is a "familiar but conceptually elusive entity" (1980, pp. 13–14). The Canadian literary scholar Northrop Frye offers us a way through this definitional dilemma. He once wrote, rather impishly, about how the plot of a piece of fiction "consists of somebody doing something" (1966, p. 33). We can take this simple insight as the core of a more comprehensive concept of story as such. Accordingly, a story is . . . *someone telling someone about somebody doing something*—a definition broad enough to embrace both fiction and fact.

For example, the someone telling could be another person or ourselves. The someone being told could, again, be another person or ourselves. The somebody doing something could also be another person or ourselves. Finally, the something being done or experienced could be an action, feeling, or thought, which in turn could be done or experienced by another person or ourselves. Armed with such an armchair analysis we may not want to advance an entire philosophy of narrative, but we can at least get started. Accordingly, four elements stand out as minimum requirements of any story (Ruth and Kenyon, 1996).

First, it is told *from* a certain *point of view*, which means we have to talk about author and narrator, and *to* a certain point of view, which means we have to talk about reader (and narrat*ee*). Second, it concerns the people who do or experience the something the story is about, which means we have to talk about *characters*, real or imagined. Third, the "something happening" that the story is about are certain events and episodes selected for telling out of all the possible events and episodes that *could* be included, then linked together in some sort of causal or sequential manner. This means we have to talk about *plot*. Fourth, we have to talk about the types of interaction between plot and character according to which stories can be catalogued, which means we must talk about *genre*.

We now consider these elements in more detail, beginning with plot. Following this, we consider the structure of the various larger stories we live within, which leads us, at the end of the chapter, to a fifth essential element of story, that of *setting*.

Plot

Every story has a plot. Plot is most obvious in the case of a murder mystery or horror thriller. Such a story keeps us on the edge of our seats, keen to know "what next?"—above all, how it turns out in the end. Plot of this type we could call *high* plot, for it is highly dramatic and highly contrived, with a carefully arranged chain of events that leads from growing conflict through thrilling climax to peaceful denouement.

But not all stories are plotted in this tight, predictable manner. Soap operas, for instance, go on and on, promising but forever postponing neat conclusions to the affairs and intrigues with which they are endlessly concerned. Though plot as such is no less at work, the satisfying finale we continually crave—with that "happily ever after" feeling we have been conditioned since childhood to desire—manages to elude us. In this way our desire is cleverly kept alive. In a more "literary" story, however, the aspect of plot is subtler, its twists and turns less obvious or abrupt, the suspense it generates less suspect, and its ending neither as predictable nor, in a sense, as integral to the structure of the story. How it turns out is not ultimately the *point* of the story. Dramatically speaking, such a story possesses a comparatively *low* plot, which emerges from within events rather than being imposed on them from above. Yet it is no less a story for this feature. Whether high or low, though, plot is the basic principle of selection, direction, and coherence that, in one philosopher's words, "*makes* events *into* a story" (Ricoeur, 1980, p. 167).

First, plot is the principle of *selection*. A story must have boundaries. It needs limits. It cannot concern everything at once. Accordingly, while certain events and episodes—certain details and dialogues—are included, others are not. As widely as some stories range in the course of unfolding, they actually *ex*clude far more than they *in*clude. Only what serves the theme, sets the mood, or advances the action is likely to be retained. All but the essential is pared away in "the sublime economy of art" (Allen, 1949, p. 156). An entire world's worth of other includable details is merely alluded to or tacitly assumed, part of the background our imagination faithfully fills in on its own. The plot is to its story, therefore, as the membrane is to its cell. It is the border of the story, what keeps things in—and out.

Second, plot is the principle of *direction*. A story must go somewhere, or at least promise to. Otherwise, we lose interest in it, not to mention faith in the storyteller. Conventionally, the direction of the story is a logical one: from first events to last, from a beginning through a middle to an end. In fact, in reading (or hearing or viewing) *any* story, it is our "sense of an ending" (Kermode, 1966) that determines how we experience both the middle and the beginning. As it were, we read the story forward but understand it backward.

This peculiar dynamic is what critic Peter Brooks calls "the anticipation of retrospection"—something he says is "our chief tool in making sense of narrative." In other words, "we read in a spirit of confidence, and also a state of dependence, that what remains to be read will restructure the provisional meanings of the already read" (1985, pp. 23, 25). To use a term coined by novelist John Gardner, our experience of a story, in reading or following it, is "profluenced" by what we conjecture lies ahead of us (1985, p. 48). If you will, the story pulls us into its own future. We literally follow the story, followability being a condition of its status *as* a story. Plot is the mechanism—what could be called the central story-*line*—by which it accomplishes this task, luring us along like the donkey pursuing the proverbial carrot, allowing us to feel that one thing is leading to another, that things are making sense, that the story has a destiny or "point."

What determines the point toward which a story unfolds is partly the *conflict* central to it. High plot or low, a story has to have conflict—subtle or obvious, physical or psychological. Whether it be within characters, between characters, or between characters and their environment, conflict is the engine of the story, what drives it toward some *goal* that effectively concludes it. Whether this goal be the solving of a mystery, the finding of a grail, the requiting of a love, or the winning of a war, its achievement is essentially what the story is "about."

Another word for conflict is the "agon" of a story (Novak, 1971). The agon is the axis on which the story turns. Hence the distinction between *prot*-agon-ists and *ant*-agon-ists. No agony at all—no trouble, as philosopher Edmund Burke has called it (Bruner, 1987)—and we would not have much of a story. If nothing goes wrong, then nothing can go right. Happy endings we tend to demand, and happy beginnings are not uncommon—as the curtain rises on a pleasant, ordinary scene, with only a hint of the trouble to come. But if we had a happy middle as well, the story would fail to satisfy. This is much of why bad news sells better than good. The principle is: no trouble, no tale; no ill, no thrill; no agon, no adventure. In sum, it is the plot that carries us from initial calm through ensuing conflict to eventual climax, conclusion, and (once more) calm. The plot thus gives the story its overall shape: narrow at the start (in terms of complexity and intensity), thicker in the middle, narrow again at the end—since everything "requires to be wound up" (Forster, 1962, p. 94).

An aspect of plot pointed to by its conflict is its implicit *morality* (Gardner, 1978). What fuels the conflict toward its resolution is the tension between a right to be upheld and a wrong to be put down, between a good to be sought and an evil to be eschewed—however little resemblance each pair bears to the code of a particular creed. In this broad way, the plot of a story mediates its meaning in both an aesthetic sense and an ethical one. A story has to have some message, however innocuous or uninspiring. Once again, stories are not innocent.

Third, plot is the principle of *coherence*. However meanderingly, a story must hang together. Its parts must, literally, cohere, and not just chronologically but causally as well. Otherwise, these same parts—the story's details and descriptions, episodes and events—seem no more connected than the items on a shopping list. To qualify as a story at all, it must amount to more than a string of *nonsequiturs*.

To the degree that a story sticks together, each part is deemed to have meaning, not in an abstract philosophical sense, or in the ethical one just considered, but *narrative* meaning, meaning within the ever-unfolding framework of the story as a whole, what the Greeks called its mythos or myth (Frye, 1988). Each detail introduced will tend to enhance our picture of a particular character or the background to the story's main action, and each event will fit or flow into a sequence of others in turn. As the story steadily unfolds into its own implicit future, fresh details and events thus possess increased potential, meaning-wise, over those that precede them. As we say, *the plot thickens*. Through the accumulation of this meaning, it renders the whole gradually greater than the sum of the parts. As it were, it makes the story both run and one.

With plot, then, we have structure and direction, morality and meaning. Without it, we have chaos and confusion. We have aimless movement and pointless activity. In a sense, we have *non*-sense. Of course, more can be said about the concept of plot than we have captured with these three elements, but we have said enough to see that if by some miracle we had a plot-less story we would have no story at all.

It is a premise of this book that if by the same miracle we had a plot-less life, then, subjectively, we would have no life at all. Composing ourselves as a more or less meaningful story in our memory and imagination—event by event, day by day, year by year—is impossible without steadily "plotting along." This emplotment is part of our response to the autobiographical imperative (as to our "fundamental project"). Moreover, it occurs both at the pre- or quasi-narrative level we spoke of in the last chapter, leading one scholar to insist on "the narrative quality of experience" itself (Crites, 1971), and at the surface or public level too. It is evident each time we undertake to talk about our lives, whether in everyday conversation or in our formal efforts at telling the story of our life overall. We need to look in more detail, then, at the place of plot in telling the stories of our lives, both individual anecdotes and the larger, longer story that lurks behind the many.

First, on the level of individual anecdotes, plot is evident in a fundamental feature of ordinary conversation: we deal in summaries. *So, what've you been up to since I saw you last?* someone might ask you. Assuming you understand that your questioner means *What have you been* doing *since I saw you last?*, how might you respond?

After you last saw me? When was that—a week ago Friday? Well, I drove home at about eleven, parked the car, unlocked the door, walked into the kitchen, made a cup of coffee, added cream from a plastic pitcher on the bottom shelf of the fridge, took two Oreo cookies out of the tin I keep in the cupboard above the stove, sat at the table sipping and eating for about 6 1/2 minutes, then felt this funny pain in my stomach, so I went to the bathroom, sat on the toilet, and . . .

How probable is this as an answer? Not very, for you would soon get the message—through a combination of throat-clearing and finger-tapping—that even though you had cut out a great deal you were still including too much. If you were to ignore these cues, you might not appreciate how you were treated. *Stop it!*, your companion might explode. *You're going into too much detail. You're wandering off track. Get to the point.* So, to avoid boring both your audience and yourself, you sort and select. You chop and cull. You edit. In fact, some of us edit our responses to such questions so fiercely, making our long stories so short, that the summary we supply says nothing about our life in the interim—simply that we are alive. *What've I been up to? Not much.*

Someone who insisted on narrating aloud their every doing and feeling—someone who in a sense had no *private* world: no inside story, only an inside-out one—would strike us as odd. "Keep it to yourself," we would counsel them for airing their self-talk so freely, "put a lid on it." We select and edit what we tell others so much that it is little surprise how much we select and edit what we tell ourselves. As we saw in Chapter 1, historians do it, and so do we, each minute of the day. What we call our memories (leastwise of events) are essentially summaries—and, as time goes by, of summaries of summaries, with ever larger chunks of our lives whizzing by memory's eye as new material presents itself for acknowledgement, analysis, and eventual transformation into memories of their own. In this manner, entire periods (or chapters) of our lives can get alluded to with only a few terse titles like *good old days* or *tough times* (Polster, 1987). Such titles hint at all the story material that lies between the lines of our lives, material that could be mined if we (or our listener) had the time to dig. To any of our stories, there is always more.

Ruthless though it be in paring down our past, such summarizing is part of plotting our lives. It is essential. How else could an autobiographer capture "the story of my life" inside a single volume? Essential or not, it is far from innocent. As Bruner puts it, our "ways of telling and the ways of conceptualizing that go with them become so habitual that they finally become recipes for structuring [our] experience itself, for laying down routes into memory" (1987, p. 31). Echoes Carolyn Heilbrun: "We tell ourselves stories of our past, make fictions or stories of it, and these narrations *become* the past, the only part of our lives that is not submerged" (1988, p. 51).

Our everyday interactions with others instruct us not only in the *degree* of summarizing we need to do, however, but also in the *kind,* in what is acceptable and important. Telling about making ourselves a coffee is acceptable, though not in such detail. Telling about going to the toilet is, in our culture at least, neither acceptable nor important—unless we are only three years old and the person questioning us is Mommy or Daddy and they are trying to get us potty-trained! In that case, information about our efforts in the bathroom is precisely what they want. The point is, importance and acceptability are not intrinsic to events themselves but functions of conventions at work in the contexts in which we recount them.

A related point is that others tend to pressure us (sometimes subtly, sometimes not) to relay summaries they will find interesting to listen to, meaning summaries—whether of situations, conversations, or events—that are not the same old story; that stick out from the norm; that go somewhere; that tell little tales with beginnings, middles, and ends, each with its dollop of conflict, its degree of suspense, and its measure of resolution (Linde, 1993; Polster, 1987). "Interesting" thus means more or less discrete story-units, not "one damned thing after another" in the annoying "and then . . . and then" manner of the ten-year-old we talked about in the last chapter. (As it were, self-editing arrives hand in hand with adulthood.)

Both aesthetically and dynamically, then, we need *conflict* in our lives—not just in terms of specific happenings that run counter to our expectations, that break with the ordinary and become to that extent recountable, but in terms of challenges that need wrestling with, interruptions that need attending to, goals that need achieving. Otherwise, we could say, our life fails to go anywhere. Fortunately, the lives of all of us are afflicted with their share of conflict, both inner and outer—whether within ourselves, between ourselves and others, or between ourselves and circumstances. (Indeed, some of us seem chronically, even deliberately, more conflicted than others!) In a sense, it is the degree and kind of conflict in our lives, plus our ways of coping with it, that render our life generally interesting in the first place, and thus worth talking about. It is partly what gives rise to our unique, personal wisdom (Randall and Kenyon, in preparation).

Both experiencing and expressing the events of our lives with a feel for their storied potential is essential to normal human living. As Polster writes, our narrative imagination seeks to frame individual "units of experience" which "heighten the sense of continual transition." Without such framing there would be no boundaries to our experience and thus "life's shape would be indiscernible, each event melting into an unimaginable oneness. A word could not exist, nor *a* meal, nor *a* day" (1987, p. 54). In order to function at all, that is, we must possess a basic level of "narrative intelligence"—both to frame our experience for ourselves and to express it meaningfully to others.

Some of us seem to possess more such "intelligence" than others, however. With uncanny (if unconscious) skill, we know how to transform even the most ordinary events into the stuff of extraordinary tales, which means we know how to draw out some details and delete others, how to pace the timing and build the suspense, how to craft a punch line and deliver it with flair, and how to use our eyes and voice for maximum effect—as in, "it's all in the telling." So it is that "stories seem to happen to people who can tell them" (Bruner, 1987, p. 12).

We must not miss the point here. On a day-to-day basis, even moment to moment, we are programmed to exclude from our attention far more than we include. Not everything that *could* make it from our outside story into our inside story *does* make it. Our very consciousness is choosey. Of "the near-infinite number of things that *could* be noticed in any given situation" (Berger, 1963, p. 56), we notice only what, for some reason, "counts." The rest, we edit out and, effectively, forget. In the next chapter we shall look at the plethora of ways we could focus on other things instead. For the moment, the question is: Why focus at all?

Why, indeed? Because psychological survival demands it. It demands it because we cannot attend to everything at once. If we tried to, we would be overwhelmed by stimuli, swamped by detail—everything compelling itself with equal force to our senses and our mind, leaving us no way to prioritize and organize the goings-on around us. To navigate our world, we have to plot our course continually—our *life*-course. Otherwise, we would run adrift and perish.

If what we notice in the present is thus restricted, then so, not surprisingly, is what we recollect from the past and project for the future. Writes David Carr (1986), "the present is only possible for us if it is framed and set off against a retained past and a potentially envisaged future" (p. 62). Continually referring what is happening in the present to what has happened in the past and may happen in the future is central to maneuvering through life. It is impossible to go through an average day without ever recalling what we did the day before or imagining what we might be doing the next—or next week, next year, or when we retire. Once again, we live according to story-time more than clock-time.

In general, we need to feel that our life is going somewhere—that on a small scale, if not a large one, the events of our life are leading to something and in that way possess a purpose or *telos*. Examples of this need abound, in fact, in the plot-talk that sprinkles everyday speech, where we routinely refer to everything from specific events to entire lives as turning out or working out or ending up in this way rather than that. In other words, we may not claim belief in a cosmic Destiny within which our personal fortunes play a predetermined part that someone, such as a psychic, is able to divine. Nor might we care to insist that everything happens for a reason, or that much in our life is meant to be—a belief even Bruner hints at in an autobiographical reference to having met someone by "ordained chance" (1983, p. 33). Yet, at a minimum, we need to feel that our being-in-the-world is not completely point*less*. In this broad fashion, all three dimensions of our life in time—our attention, memory, and imagination—are "emplotted."

Plot also patterns our action in the world. In the words of Carr again, "we are constantly striving . . . to occupy the story-teller's position with respect to our own actions." Indeed, unstoried action in the present is impossible; narrative is "intertwined with the course of life." Carr's conclusion is that stories "are told in being lived and lived in being told" (1986, pp. 60–62). His perspective is echoed by Richard Ochberg (1995). In an article entitled "Life Stories and Storied Lives," Ochberg argues that "individuals do not merely tell stories, after the fact, about their experiences; instead they live out their affairs in storied forms" (p. 116). In his view, there is "a structure to sequences of lived action that is similar to the structure of a traditional plot" (p. 116). Thus, people "*perform* their lives in storied form" (p. 117).

Finally, plot is a continual component of the composition of our entire life-course. While many of us keep trying to plan the shape of our life, others of us have the feeling it is unfolding on its own, by emergent design—as Bateson puts it, "following an underlying grammar and an evolving aesthetic" (1989, p. 3). And as it unfolds it gets more complicated, thickened (sometimes unnecessarily) by the people, projects, and problems of which it is more and more comprised.

Not only does our life-course thicken, however, but it twists and turns as well. We can illustrate this with an exercise often assigned us in a counseling context, when asked to graph a life-line to trace the highs and lows of our lives thus far. At the nadir of the lows and the apex of the highs we identify the major turning points in our path: the birth of a child, the completion of a degree, the death of a spouse. Looking at our own lives, it may be difficult to see the sweep of the story-line these turning points trace. It can be easier to pick it out in others' lives instead, for even in the case of those closest to us we experience others' lives always at a distance, outside-in—especially after they have died. This helps explain our enduring attraction to biographies, for in such works the overall shape of a person's life-in-time is made to stand out with satisfying (if largely fictional) clarity.

Literary critic Wayne Booth (1988) invites us, for instance, to list "all the life-plot summaries" we can think of. "Though our stories are unique," he writes, "they fall into 'genres' [see Frye's 'modes'] that are obviously not infinite in number" (p. 289). Tongue-in-cheek, he gives us his list of these limited genres: "from high promise to happiness to misery; from beginning misery to happiness to misery; from misery to misery to maximum misery . . . ; from happiness to happiness to misery; from happiness to happiness to higher happiness . . . ; from promise to promise to sudden accidental death. And so on" (p. 289). We shall come back to such matters soon, for they point to the issue of different genres of stories overall, which have to do with the ways in which plot is entwined with character.

Character

Once we accept that life is inseparable from lifestory, we are bound to look through the lenses of typical story categories, among which character is key. A story has to have characters. Whether the story be fiction or "faction" (Steele, 1986), someone has to do or endure whatever it is "about."

The first thing to realize is that a character in a story is not a real person, merely the impression of one evoked by the words of an author or the images of a camera. As for the blanks these words and images leave, we fill them in on our own. However, such filling-in is essential to our dealings not just with fictional persons but with real ones as well. Meaningful interaction with our fellow human beings is possible at all because of our capacity to *imagine* what their lives are like beyond what we can see of them directly—both their physical existence (where they live and what they eat when they go home) and their inner experience (what they think and how they feel when they are by themselves). Thus, life imitates art. That is, our everyday challenge is the same as the novelist's. Writes literary scholar Percy Lubbock, "we are continually piecing together our fragmentary evidence about the people around us and moulding their images in thought. It is the way in which we make our world; partially, imperfectly, very much at haphazard, but still perpetually, everybody deals with his experience like an artist" ([1921] 1965, p. 7).

Put another way, we never deal with other people *as they are*, in their completeness. Indeed, we could not. (We can scarcely deal with ourselves in this respect!) We see a body in front of us, a human being more or less similar to ourselves, and yet as to what he or she feels, how he or she sees the world, and how he or she became who he or she is—this is essentially a mystery. What we know about another person is based on guesswork. It amounts to an accumulation of impressions related to memories (stories, versions) of previous encounters and to fantasies (or prejudices) projected onto him or her from the depths of our own experience. If we ignored what we *think* we know and tried to be receptive to all the person *is*, we would be unable to function. As novelist Somerset Maugham says, "We know very little even of the persons we know most intimately . . . [They] are too elusive, too shadowy . . . too incoherent and contradictory" (1938, p. 133).

Just as we can get by with only summaries of events, so we can get by with only summaries of people. In the last chapter, we called these summaries storyotypes. Though the storyotypes we form of some, such as those we know most intimately, are more lifelike and flexible than those we form of others, the drive holds steady to form them nonetheless. It is the *biographical* imperative. We can relate to others only by characterizing them, often rather crudely. Either we idolize them—put them on a pedestal—or we villainize them—focus on their less flattering side, perhaps the side that most struck us when we formed our first impressions. Even without going to such extremes, our pictures of others are seldom completely fair (though, again, our maturity is measured by our willingness to subject them to revision, to be open to new sides that new situations evoke).

Witness our habit of misrepresenting what others have said or done when we are reporting an encounter with them to someone else. We paraphrase their words with our own; we distort the tone and exaggerate the accent they actually used; we substitute our gestures for theirs. In fact, how we portray other people (and thus relate to them) says less about them than about us—our needs, our self-concept, our unresolved conflicts and unfulfilled dreams. If you will, they are characters in *our* lifestory (as we are in theirs)—members of the "community of internalized others" that each of us is (Parry and Doan, 1994, p. 5). As such, they are transformed from real people in their own right to fictional ones in inevitably storyotyped form. In retelling an encounter with them, we place emphasis where it might not have been originally and cast our own behavior in ways that flatter or vindicate us but may make fools of them, depending on who we are trying to impress with what version of what took place. Further evidence of this biographical imperative are our descriptions of certain individuals as "characters"—whether interesting or comical or weird—or, if especially unusual, as *real* characters.

Characters in fiction are either major or minor, a distinction that concerns the agency a character possesses in how the plot unfolds. Major characters are critical to the development of the story, while minor ones merely support major ones or else are expendable extras, nice to include but, strictly speaking, unnecessary to the plot. A second distinction is between "round" characters and "flat" ones (Forster, 1962). Flat characters (which can in turn be major or minor) are "simple, two-dimensional, endowed with very few traits, highly predictable in behaviour" (Prince, 1987, p. 12). We call them "stock." They are uninteresting for their own sake, but are simply instruments by which the plot is carried along. Round characters, in contrast, are "complex, multi-dimensional, capable of surprising behaviour" (p. 12). Their character can change; it develops. In fact, it is the development (or building) of character with which serious fiction is usually most concerned.

But just as the full reality of others is regularly lost on us, so is the full reality of ourselves. In our own imagination, we are frequently far flatter than we are in actuality. Moreover, the impression we hold of ourselves— what we are like, how we look—often bears an ambiguous relationship to the impressions held of us by others. Plus, it can change: one day (or hour) wildly inflated relative to "reality," and wholly *de*flated the next. As we saw in the last chapter, depending on the story-lines stimulated within us and the emotions they trigger, we can see ourselves as wizard in one situation and worm in another. Indeed, from saint to sinner, hero to victim, genius to dunce, winner to loser: the range of images we can entertain of ourselves— what McAdams calls "imagoes" (1988)—is so wide that we could be said to suffer from "multiphrenia" (Gergen, 1991, pp. 77–80). None of us is one person alone. Says novelist Norman Brown, "every person . . . is many persons; a multitude made into one person; a corporate body . . . a corporation" (Parry and Doan, 1994, p. 5).

Just as we character-ize others, so we continually (if not consistently) character-ize ourselves. Self-*concept* means self-characterization. Whenever I tell someone about something I did (or that happened to me), the "I" who did the something (or the "me" to whom it happened) is not the same "I" who does the telling. The latter is the narrator; the former, a character in the narrator's tale, a necessarily simplified version—caricature, really— of the actual "I" involved in the initial event. My motives at the time were more mixed than can now be recalled; the precise nature of my thoughts and feelings then is, in retrospect, lost.

The term character has long held an honored place in the history of thought as an *ethical* term. We think of a person's character as the core of virtues constant throughout their lives. To use character as an *aesthetic* term may seem therefore a novel approach. But it has long been a *theatrical* term too. As such, it is pivotal to appreciating the poetics of composing a life, from childhood on.

As children, we tend to *pre*-tend. Pretending is—or has been, till the advent of TV—a large part of childhood play. Sneaking around the alleys of our town, we are spies behind enemy lines. Playing catch on the front lawn, we are champion atheletes in a World Series showdown. Building some thingamajig out of junk from the garage, we are NASA engineers designing an interstellar probe. Dressing up in adult clothes, we are Mommy and Daddy playing house. Pretending is central to becoming ourselves. Nor does it cease with adolescence.

In adolescence, we can be intent on imitating a certain look, either to fit in or to stand out (or both at once); thus, we mimic trends set by rock stars and other idols, by the "in"-gang or "cool" crowd. They present various personae that we try on for size, trading them in and up as cooler ones appear. Thus, largely unconsciously, we patch together a persona-lity. Indeed, such "play-acting with characters or characteristics," says Wayne Booth, "is one of the main ways that we build what becomes our character" (1988, p. 252). We grow into what began as an act.

With adulthood, this tendency becomes more covert. However, while we may no longer indulge ourselves in games of make-believe, as in childhood, or scramble to be part of "the scene," as in adolescence, we delude ourselves if we think we thereby rely on our own aesthetic resources for composing our lives. The need to keep up appearances (or keep up with the Joneses) does not so soon vanish. Indeed, how many of our adult activities did we not first get into because of the look they enabled us to exude or the crowd they allowed us to join? More or less consciously, we continue wearing masks, projecting an everchanging series of personae to either meet, manage, or manipulate the impressions that others inevitably form (Goffman, 1959). From our parents to our pals, from actors in movies to ads in magazines, we take our cues as to how to walk and talk, dress and behave, then gradually weave these habits into our own peculiar costume.

That all the world is thus a stage is more obvious in some corners than in others. In business or politics, for example, pretension seems everything, appearance all. (What self-respecting leader would dare go forth without a personal "image consultant"?) While to most people there is usually much more behind their masks, more than meets our eye, in the case of others there can be so much less. Their whole manner seems studied; their voice, calculated to impress; their gestures, grand. Sensing this can lead us to a general cynicism about social interaction, never quite trusting the "acts" of others, always wanting to peek behind the scenes and get the *real* story.

But even the sincerest among us, in our most ordinary activities and intimate encounters, can be said to be playing to an audience, putting on an act—if only the act of pretending we are not putting on an act! If we ignored our audience completely (where they are coming from, what they will understand), if we spoke our own private language, behaved according to our own code, we would soon be deemed insane. Indeed, amid a crowd of strangers or totally alone, we are frequently still on stage, our audience merely some internalized Other—whether a deceased parent, a Divine Judge, a fantasy companion, or a mob of admiring fans. At the very least (as sociologists will tell us), we live much of our lives in terms of roles, which, however much we adapt them to what we think is uniquely us, are prescribed by our profession, scripted by our family, and assigned by the culture and gender to which we belong.

In short, none of us is as original as we assume. What we consider our unique personality is, in a sense, a composite of the personae by which we act. While our peculiar composition is unique to us, its components can be "stock." Says Wayne Booth, however, it is only through the continuous process of "embracing and sloughing off successive 'characters' " that we each "produce a life story that is uniquely 'my own' " (pp. 288–289). As it were, the road to who we are is paved with good (or bad) pretensions!

Arising from this are a number of questions. How does each of us characterize ourselves in the midst of the stories we relate? What roles do we (perceive ourselves to) play in the midst of our acts in the dramas of daily life? As what sorts of character do we see ourselves—major or minor, flat or round? As flat in some roles (e.g., as employee) but round in others (e.g., as bowler, lover, mother)? And how have our particular personae, plus our characterizations of others, taken their cue from the larger stories by which we are shaped—above all, the family into which we were born? Finally, if, as we are seeing, our characterizations of ourselves can be as numerous as the versions of our life's events, then, ultimately, who am "I"? What, after all, is the story of *my* life?

Such questions concern the familiar notion of self-*concept*—of how we *see* ourselves. By thinking of self-concept in terms of self-characterization, however, we give it a more aesthetic and dynamic twist. Not only that, but we shift the ground on which we base our understanding of human nature— from one dominated by social science to one shared more equally with the humanities and arts.

Genre

Character is entwined with plot. In the celebrated query of Henry James, "what is character but the determination of incident? What is incident but the illustration of character?" The coincidence of character and plot applies in *life*story too. Just as we shape events in our life through our choices and decisions, so events shape us. We need only ask someone who has lived through a famine or war. Says Joseph Campbell, "our life evokes our character. You find out more about yourself as you go on" (Campbell and Moyers, 1988, p. 130).

Northrop Frye (1988) offers a schema for appreciating the broad ways in which character and plot interact, each with its deep structure and its narrative conventions. Accordingly, if we classify stories in relation to "the hero's power of action" vis-à-vis both the other characters and the surrounding environment (natural and social), then "there are a limited number of possible ways of telling a story" (p. 54), or, as it were, storying styles. Insofar as that power of action "may be greater than ours, less, or roughly the same," Frye outlines five main modes of fiction: *myth*, *romance*, *tragedy*, *comedy*, and *irony*.

With myth, the hero is superior *in kind* to all other characters and to us, as well as to the environment—just as are heroes in stories of gods and goddesses. With romance, the hero is superior to all other characters, and to us, not in kind but *in degree*. Heroes' actions are marvelous but still human, as with the heroes of high adventure so common on the silver screen, who rise above all odds to defeat the dragon or put down the evil or save the day (see Zweig, 1974). With tragedy, heroes are superior in degree both to other characters and to us, but not to their natural or moral environment, which accounts for their eventual undoing—MacBeth and Lear being classic examples. With comedy, the hero is superior neither to others nor to the environment but rather is one of us. With fiction of the ironic mode, the hero is inferior to us in both power and intelligence, which means "we have the sense of looking down on a scene of bondage, frustration, or absurdity" (Frye, 1966, pp. 23–24).

To this list, James Hillman adds a sixth: *picaresque*. Picaresque is a blend of tragedy, comedy, and romance. "Its central figure"—epitomized by Cervantes's character Don Quixote—"does not develop (or deteriorate), but goes through episodic, discontinuous movements. His narrative ends abruptly without achievement for there is no goal; so the denouement can neither be the resolution of comedy nor the fatal flaw of tragedy" (1975, p. 141).

Applying these modes—or genres—to lived lives might seem to be straining unfairly to see parallels between literature and life. But more than a few narrative psychologists have employed them thus (see Keen, 1986; McAdams, 1988; Murray, 1989), guided by the conviction that if the idea of lifestory has integrity at all, then allowance must be made not just for character and plot but for *genre* as well.

In "Life as Narrative," Jerome Bruner (1987) speculates on "the forms of self-telling" (p. 16), a phrase he elsewhere uses synonomously with genres. In an article coauthored with Susan Weisser, he says that "the shape of a life is as much a function of the conventions of genre and style in which it is couched as it is . . . of what happened in the course of that life" (1991, p. 129). A decade and a half before, Hillman had stressed a similar point: "The way we imagine our lives is the way we are going to go on living our lives. For the manner in which we tell ourselves what is going on is the genre through which events become experiences" (1975, p. 146). To repeat our point in Chapter 2, stories consist of ideas, emotions, *and* actions.

In their own reflections on genre in personal narratives, Kenneth and Mary Gergen (1983, 1984) ask whether there are "commonly shared rules that limit how it is we can communicate about life across time? What are the boundaries," they inquire, "within which one can make sense to one's fellow creatures?" (1984, p. 174). Starting from their conviction that we render intelligible the events of our lives "by locating them in a sequence or 'unfolding process' . . . the sensible sequence of ongoing stories" (p. 174), they go on to consider "the varieties of narrative form . . . that arrange a sequence of events as they pertain to the achievement of a particular goal state." Their conclusion is that there are only three "prototypical or primitive narrative forms: those in which progress toward the goal is enhanced, those in which it is impeded, and those in which no change occurs." They call these three forms, respectively, the stability narrative, the progressive narrative, and the regressive narrative.

"Theoretically," say the Gergens, "one may envision a potential infinity of variations on these rudimentary forms. However, for reasons of social utility, aesthetic desirability, and cognitive capability, the culture may limit itself to a truncated repertoire of possibilities" (1984, p. 176). A progressive narrative followed by a regressive narrative is what we call *tragedy*. *Comedy* is the opposite, a regressive narrative followed by a progressive one. *Romance* is a series of progressive-regressive phases. These basic narrative forms, they say, "serve to structure one's personal accounts" (p. 177). Moreover, they may structure the way we *hear* such accounts as well. Early on, we learn to recognize people's propensities in both telling and living, and so to pick out the optimist from the pessimist, the joker from the sourpuss, the adventurer from the tragedian.

Extending our options still more in this regard, and lending empirical support to the range of self-genres to which people live, is the work of Ruth and Oberg (1996) on "ways of life" among Scandinavian seniors. Based on extensive interviews, they identified six self-images in terms of which their subjects have constructed their lives: *the suffering one, the loser, the fighter, the altruist, the careerist,* and *the happy one.*

Whether we limit our list of life-genres to three or five or six, explicit in such schemas—which are schemas of storying styles—are two ideas that need modifying if we are going to use them in relation to lifestory. The first is the very idea of hero. The second is that these genres can be found in pure form.

As for the first, sometimes we may not feel much like the hero in our own lifestory—in the sense not of "heroic" even, but simply of "agent of action" vis-à-vis others and our environment. This is the sense in which the term is used by Carol Pearson (1989). In *The Hero Within*, Pearson analyses five main archetypes by which people orient themselves amid their relationships and their world—as either orphan, martyr, warrior, wanderer, or magician. But even with this more general sense of the term, applying "hero" to ourselves can feel unjustified.

Other personalities and powers can so dominate us that we feel pushed to the background of the drama of our own lives. Such a dilemma has traditionally been the plight of the poor more than the rich of the world, and of women more than men. In Pearson's view, for instance, women are conditioned from the beginning into the martyr mode, to living their lives in service to others. As one of our colleagues once remarked, during the nine years she was married she felt that not she but her husband was the main character in *her* lifestory. But gender is not automatically a factor. The poignant words of David Copperfield at the beginning of Dickens's novel articulate a concern that can weigh upon us all: "whether I shall turn out to be the hero of my own life or whether that station will be held by anybody else, these pages must show."

The degree we feel ourselves to be the hero of our own lifestory can thus vary greatly and can change (as can our mood) from day to day. Some days, our spirit soars because we feel we are the primary agent in determining our life: the master of our destiny and captain of our fate. Other days, a sense of powerlessness prevails. In charge, it appears, are forces and factors beyond our control. Our *locus* of control is external, not internal, to ourselves.

As for the second idea, these modes of fiction are rarely found alone. Popular as they are in the construction of events in our everyday world—witness familiar headline formulas like *Heroic action saves drowning teen* or *Weekend adventure turns to tragedy*—a movie or novel run along tightly genre-ated lines might be too predictable for our taste. However much we may want literature to imitate life, in life things are never so neat; the modes are continually mixed.

The events of any given day, as we *perceive* and construct them, can shift amusingly from one genre to another. First, the car refuses to start (minor tragedy), then we win a bowling ball in the office lottery (comedy), then the boss gives us an exciting new assignment (adventure), then our ex-husband sprains an ankle jogging with his new girlfriend (irony). Of course, such genre-mixing also operates on a level less mundane. "While one part of me knows the soul goes to death in tragedy," says Hillman, "another is living a picaresque fantasy, and a third engaged in the heroic comedy of improvement" (1989, p. 81).

Such variety is familiar to us if we have ever once got a sense of our "social psyche" (Booth, 1988, p. 252), of the bewildering complexity of our inner world and its "multiphrenic" state. Indeed, most of us take it for granted that we have several "sides"—a realization on which some psychologists have in fact built a theory of "*sub*-personalities." Each "sub," say its advocates, has its own developmental history, its own way of characterizing us, its own emotional agenda, and its own way of plotting—or *sub*-plotting—the course of our life (Vargiu, 1978). Moreover, each is evoked by some of the people we deal with more than by others, which helps explain why with certain individuals we can feel light and cheery, while with others, heavy or sad. This internal cast of characters may make the line rather fine, then, between the normal diversity to which all are inclined and the *ab*-normal division that is the signal not of sub- but of *multiple* personality.

Point of View

Every story has a point of view. In literary terms, however, point of view does not mean an opinion or a philosophy, at least in the way it does in everyday speech. (As we have noted, no story is without bias: there is always a point, an agenda, a message.) Rather, point of view refers to the construction of a story in terms of the angle from which it is told. The point is, a story is always told; it does not come from nowhere. The same applies with *life*story. As narrators of our own narratives, we each have our ways of self-telling.

The concept of point of view is as complicated as any we shall encounter in literary theory. It concerns, among other things, the perspective from which the events of the story are portrayed. In terms of "the rhetoric of fiction" (Booth, 1966), at least four such perspectives need factoring in: that of the author, the narrator, the protagonist (character or characters), and the reader. (Other theorists have fine-tuned this list by adding such distinctions as real author and implied author, real and implied reader, and narratee.) From each perspective, we effectively have a different story. The story as experienced by the author (out of whose imagination it has come) is not exactly the same as that portrayed by the narrator (who may be unreliable to some degree); nor as it would be from the perspective of a character *in* the story; nor, certainly, as it is experienced by the reader. Literature teachers use this insight to illustrate how the same story instantly becomes a different story when told from a different point of view. Think how our sense of a favorite novel might change if it were narrated not as it is (say, by a detached, omniscient narrator) but in some other manner instead: by a main character, a minor character, by ourself (as reader), by a woman instead of a man.

Such distinctions invite us to see how, rhetorically, ordinary self-consciousness is an extraordinary matter—how, in a sense, we possess several selves at once: self-as-author, self-as-narrator, self-as-protagonist, and self-as-reader. As we shall see in the next chapter, central to taking more authority for our lives (and in that sense restorying them) is looking at our life from a different point of view—which means from the perspective of a different self: self-as-author, for example, rather than self-as-reader looking on passively from the outside, or self-as-character caught fatefully amid the action. In this way, we loosen ourselves at least a little from the usual ways we interpret the events of our lives—enough to open ourselves to experiment with *new* ways.

For the remainder of this section, we shall confine our focus to the perspective of self-as-narrator. Accordingly, there are at least four aspects of self-narration that, as we listen for them in *how* people tell themselves, clue us to the existential angle from which they experience their lifestories. They are *time, tone, vocabulary*, and *voice*.

Before considering these aspects, we must remember that they apply to written stories and filmed ones alike, for even when an actual voice periodically breaks in to tell the story, the eye of the camera is the functional equivalent of the narrator's point of view. Once we appreciate this parallel, watching films for subtle differences in camerawork becomes a fascinating enhancement of our moviegoing pleasure. For example, an odd-angled Hitchcock camera style mediates a much different mood to the events it depicts from the a panoramic perspective capturing the same events under the direction of Cecil B. DeMille.

Time

Most stories are narrated in the past tense: *It was a dark and stormy night*, or *He said, she said* . . . Nowadays, however, we increasingly find stories narrated in the present tense. Few, though, will be told in the future tense—except in weather reports, economic forecasts, or prophetic texts: *And it shall come to pass that* . . . As in literature, so in life: the same options pertain. While in everyday conversation past tense prevails, it is curiously common to hear obviously past occurrences narrated in the present tense: *And then I go* . . . , *and she goes.* . . . Yet, future tense is common too, since as narrators of our own lives, much of which we still have to live, we are frequently involved in anticipating what we are *going* to do: *Tomorrow, I hope to* . . . *When I retire, I plan to.* . . . Taking such distinctions seriously, we begin to notice that, timewise, people tend to be oriented to their lifestory material in individual ways. Where some seem to live in the past, others are focused on the present. Still others appear bored with the present and impatient with its petty pace; their talk is characteristically future talk.

Tone

What literature teachers are keen for students to appreciate is the peculiar tone that characterizes a given author's work. A subtle feature, not readily noticed, it is nonetheless real. One novel is narrated in what to a twentieth-century ear sounds high and formal, as if snootily detached from the events it recounts; another's, in a manner down-to-earth, even coarse. Of course, countless gradations lie between such extremes—from sweet to sarcastic, angry to ironic, questioning to cocky, flat to melodramatic, holier-than-thou to humbler-than-all.

With a slight stretch of imagination, however, we can pick out corresponding varieties in the "narrative tone" of the people we meet each day (McAdams, 1996). While some are attributable to the accent of the region from which they hail, others are more individual in nature. Certain people's words are uttered with a staunch "I told you so" always behind them or "what's the world coming to!"; for others, "it's not *my* fault" or "Nobody bothered to ask *me*." For others, it is a question: "Does what I say make any sense?" For others still, it is "From where I sit atop my high tower, looking out over the world and its mundane affairs . . . " For others: "woe is me" or "life's done me wrong."

Vocabulary

Tied to tone are the actual words a narrator employs. Differences in vocabulary are obvious in literature: Hemingway has a different way with words from Hardy's or Atwood from Oates'. However, such differences are scarcely less obvious when it comes to people's everyday speech, once we learn to listen for them. Accordingly, some have a penchant for expressing themselves in vague generalities, rarely getting to what *we* think ought to be the point. Similarly, some have a predilection for obscure metaphors, flowery circles, or high-sounding jargon, while others stick to short, simple words and a no-nonsense way of arranging them. Of course, many such differences are due to our education level, our "linguistic intelligence" (see Gardner, 1990), or simply our audience. We would not use the same vocabulary in talking to a six-year-old as to a Ph.D. in philosophy, or to an eighty-year-old who is hard of hearing.

Voice

"Voice" is really a meta-concept, embracing all three aspects we have just outlined, but it has at least two related meanings. In political terms, as we indicated in Chapter 2, it points to the issue of personal power (see Gilligan, 1982), particularly of "finding our own voice" in the course of assuming the authorship of our lives. In poetical-grammatical terms, though, it refers to such specific distinctions as that between active and passive ways of expressing a point, or between the indicative, imperative, and subjunctive moods. It also refers to basic features like volume, emphasis, and drama in the actual *sound* of what someone says.

For example, some habitually use active linguistic constructions, as in *I did, I am, I will*. Others show a preference for passive ones, giving the impression that it is not so much that they *do* things as that things *happen to* them: *It happened to me that . . .* or *I was forced to . . .* or *they're going to make me . . .* Wordwise, they place themselves in a passive position vis-à-vis what is going on around them—like a woman in one of our classes whose telltale phrase in relating her lifestory was *somehow I managed*. "Somehow I managed," she would sigh, "to get my degree, raise three children, survive cancer," and so on. To her astonished classmates, her voice portrayed her as someone *to* whom events occur—as, in effect, the victim, an *anti*-hero, not the agent who *causes* events or *makes* things happen by her own powers. People with this orientation on the world might make frequent reference to an anonymous "they" who are constantly calling the shots. In part, of course, such an orientation may be a function of gender. As Ruth and Vilkko (1996) note, for instance, in their study of Scandinavian seniors, "women often use 'we' instead of 'I' when describing how their lives evolved", and "describe themselves as objects rather than subjects in their lives" (p. 170).

Gender trend or not, in a sense one's voice tells all. A characteristically self-deprecating voice says: *I don't matter. My life is uninteresting and unimportant.* A more authoritative (perhaps actually louder) voice communicates something quite different, as does that of someone who fills his or her speech with phrases like *I showed him* or *I told them off.* However, all such differences are not just interesting, not inconsequential features of the sounds that roll off a person's lips, but critical indicators of their storying style, of the ways, rhetorically, they compose their lives.

THE LARGER STORIES WE LIVE WITHIN

We do not compose our lives in a vacuum. If it were possible to do so, perhaps we might *think* we would be freer to be who we are, and could see and experience others as they are too. In reality, the dividing line between our own lifestories and those of others can be very fine. Parents sometimes "live through" their children, for example, and children often "live out" their parents' dreams. More profoundly than this, our individual repertoire of story material, our characteristic storying style, and the shape of our lifestory overall—all have been deeply influenced by the several social systems in which we have had involvement throughout our life, or in which we have lived, like it or not, as fish live in water.

These systems, which correspond to the social, structural, and interpersonal dimensions of lifestory we discussed in Chapter 2, are what one psychologist refers to as "cultures of embeddedness" (see Kegan, 1982). We can think of each as a *larger story* within which our personal one is set. Together, they constitute the ever-changing *con*text within which we weave our lives.

We call such systems stories not to minimize their tangible reality—though, because we are "in" them, we can never see them set apart from us *as stories* in the way we can movies or novels—but to underline the fact that ultimately all we know of them, as of other people, is in terms of our interpretation or *experience* of them. And our experience of them is based on information and anecdotes we have heard and internalized from others, and/or tell ourselves, about where these story-systems have come from, where they are going, and what they are like. Moreover, our situation in each is analagous to that of the people inside a novel. We are a particular character (flat or round), playing a particular role (major or minor), contributing a particular *sub*plot to its unfolding drama.

Examples of larger stories include, first, a *family story*. As our first culture, the family makes known "its norms and mores . . . through family stories" with which, on some level, we are "always in conversation" (Stone, 1988, p. 7f). However, not only does our family *have* stories but, like each of us, *is* a story. Says Thomas Moore in *Care of the Soul*: "when we talk about family, we are talking about the characters and themes that have woven together to form our identities." In other words, "that personal family, which seems so concrete, is always an imaginal entity" (1992, p. 32).

To appreciate this imaginal aspect, we need only ask our parents or siblings about their respective experiences within our family, or what memories of it are central for them, and we can wonder whether we even grew up in the same household! What each of us has internalized as "my family" seems a figment of our imagination. Of course, the situation is often complicated by the fact that many of us belong to more than one family in the course of our life. Besides the family into which we were born can be our adopted or elected family as well, the one we blend into if a parent remarries or produce for ourselves by having children of our own.

Beyond our family story, on the large end of the spectrum, is our *clan story*—for example, that of the Kenyon tribe or the Randall bunch, with roots spreading centuries deep and continents wide. On the small end of the spectrum is a *couple story*, which is what gets composed in the course of any close relationship—whether friendship, romance, or marriage. As William Bridges stresses, "To become a couple is to agree implicitly to live in terms of another's story, although it sometimes takes time to get the part down really well" (1980, p. 71). Living in terms of each other's lifestories, a common story develops between us. (Between you and me is a "we," a mutual reference with a life of its own, greater than the sum of its parts.) Though each of us will experience it and tell it according to our own version, it is composed of all the times we have shared, conversations we have enjoyed, conflicts we have endured, and dreams we have dreamed. It is thus itself a narrative text, with plot-lines to be identified and themes to be read.

Then there is a *community story*—or stories, as the case can be for many in our mobile age. A community story is the lifestory of the particular neighborhood or village, town or city, into which we are born, in which we grow up, or in which we reside. As sociologist David Flynn (1991) puts it, "personal stories blend into, are chapters within, community stories" (p. 25). That is, no one is an island: "as an individual, I have my own story, but if I am not a character in a *community*-story, then it is difficult to imagine what I am doing now, what I intend to do" (p. 25). In Flynn's view, we can even "classify . . . communities by their stories" (p. 33). By "story" here, though, Flynn means not so much the *history* of the community, which is the story told *about* it, outside-in. Rather, he means the myth it tells itself, inside and inside-out, about what it has been in the past, what it is like in the present, and what will happen to it in the future. This myth will in turn have its unique spirit, whether of despair about the passing of a bygone day, or of hope—of things moving onward and upward (see Owen, 1987).

A community can be understood in a formal sense as a political unit—like a village, state, or nation—or in the informal sense of any group of people with whom we relate over a significant period, with whose fortunes our own are entwined. So defined, it could include a support group, the participants in a weekend retreat, a gang of friends in a college dorm, a regiment of soldiers with whom we fight a war, or a network of colleagues with whom we share a discipline. In any one, of course, we can conceivably form much tighter and more lasting bonds than we do with the members of our own family.

Everyone is part of a family story, a clan story, at least a few couple stories, and a number of community stories, too. But most of us become involved in other types as well. There is a *company story* (or corporate story), for example, in which, as employees, we play a unique role but share a common structure and, in principle, a common goal. Also, there can be a *club story* (or two), meaning the association we have over time with members of the same sports team, hobby group, or service organization. In such involvements, our fortunes are thrown in with those of people we might not otherwise encounter except in pursuit of the interest we share. One kind of club story is a *profession story*—the one in which we participate with all other lawyers or nurses, teachers or truckers, by practicing the same trade. At staff parties, union meetings, or professional conferences, it gets retold and reaffirmed.

A *creed story* is a type of larger story, too. Creed stories are the grand "master narratives" in which our lifestories fit because we are born into or espouse the same philosophy or beliefs. Examples include the Roman Catholic story, the Islamic story, and the communist story. As we consider in the following chapter, being involved in either of these schools us in a particular version of the world (though it is proclaimed to us not as a story but as simply "the truth")—of how it began, what it is like, where it is going;

its recurring conflicts, its key players; who we are in the midst of it and what we ought to be doing. For "as long as the Christian story was dominant in the Western World," says one source, "people were able to live their lives intentionally by experiencing themselves as characters within that story and interpreting events in their lives in terms of the meaning provided by Christianity's dramatic and cosmic events" (Parry and Doan, 1994, p. 6). Within each such story, we also learn a set of sayings that witness to the frame of reference within which we make sense of our lives: sayings like "Thank God" or "the will of Allah" or "blessing" or "karma" or "power to the people." Usually, these stories are mediated within smaller groups in turn—such as congregations or cell groups (each with its own *community story*)—where their grip on our imagination is regularly reinforced through lectures, rituals, and sermons.

A still larger story that shapes our lives is the *culture story* that we were born into or have come to adopt. "Culture" is a vast concept. A discussion of it quickly opens into a consideration of such variations as dominant culture, counterculture, or subculture; as high culture versus popular culture; or as urban versus rural. Though the word can refer to such specific things as customs or lifestyle, aesthetics or ethics, we use it here in the broad, everyday sense in which, for example, Western culture is different from Native culture, or Chicano from Caribbean culture, or French from English. Such differences are not merely historical or political in nature, of course, but frequently linguistic as well, having to do with the very language people speak, with how its grammar and deep structure uniquely dertermine their experience of the world.

Related to culture story, then, is the *class story* in which we grew up and from which many of our dearest precepts derive. For example, though such distinctions may be unfashionable, upper class people (economically speaking) generally inhale a different air and enjoy a different existence than do those of the middle or lower class.

Also related is the country or *national story*. The American story, for instance, is different from the Canadian one, with a unique chain of events to which its citizens must in some way be oriented insofar as they self-identify *as* Americans: the Civil War, the bombing of Pearl Harbor, the death of JFK, and so on. These events are, in a sense, part of every American's lifestory, the content it must take into account. As such, they correspond to what gerontologists call period effects.

A variation on the national story can be the *political story*, the particular version of our collective past, present, and future that a given party will expound at election time and enact when in power. In addition is the *generation story* of which we are part as members of the same "cohort"—for example, whether we grew up during the Depression or at the outbreak of the Cold War; the *race story* in which we are rooted, with its own long saga behind it; and, finally and most profoundly, the *gender story* of which, genetically and biologically, we are unquestionably part.

Naturally, the various levels of these larger stories will interact, overlap, and frequently conflict, cradling our individual lives in roughly concentric fashion—the family story within the clan story within the community story, and so on. That is, we live within stories within stories within stories; in fact, within many at once. The lines that divide them are generally fine. For instance, the members of a support group or church clique can sometimes feel more like brothers and sisters than can our own siblings. As well, through intermarriage, clan stories are frequently interwoven within—and thus form the fabric of—community stories, especially in rural areas and small towns. Such observations underline that a full explanation of the construction, complexity, and inter(textual)connection of each of these larger social systems *as stories* is beyond our mandate here. Yet while such an explanation is more fitting for a book on sociology or history, it is still relevant to the subject of this one. Obviously, the larger story-world by which a person is shaped and in relation or reaction to which they *re*-story will be significantly different for a white, Protestant, rural, middle-class North American male born in the 1920s than for a nonwhite, upper class, suburban, Middle Eastern female born in the 1970s, and so on. Both psychologically and sociologically, we live in different story-worlds.

Concerning larger stories in general, however, three points are relevant to the storying of our lives: *poetic structure, narrative environment*, and *coauthoring*.

Poetic Structure

Each system in which we are rooted has its own *life*story, and thus a unique poetic structure. By this is meant it has its own history, with chroniclers (official and unofficial) thereof, and its own levels—outside, inside, inside-out, and outside-in. Also, like any story, it can be analyzed in terms of its characters, points of view, and themes; its style and atmosphere; its guiding genre and spirit (see Owen, 1987); its critical turning points; its tensions, conflicts, and (thus) morality. It can be analyzed in terms of its own plot lines, too—that is, what events and details get excluded and included in ordinary narrating within it, what activities count as important or acceptable, what makes sense and what does not, where things are going or *ought* to go, and finally who is generally *inside* its story-world and who is not. (In other words, it implicitly divides the world into "us and them.") Furthermore, it can be analyzed in terms of its unique brand of drama.

For example, the overall *plot* of the generation story of the late 1930s to mid-1940s of this century could be said to have been driven by the conflict between the Axis and Allied powers. No matter whose side the media supported, good and evil were rendered easy to distinguish and the moral choice made clear. Moreover, the central characters in the *theater* of war were obvious to all, as either heroes (Churchill and McArthur) or villains (Hitler and Hirohito). And a very dramatic story it all made, both at the time and in history books since—lots of action, lots of suspense, lots of pathos; much more dramatic than the saga of World War I, with its localized trench battles and perpetual *tug* of war.

Closer to home, when each of us is born we are pulled into the unfolding story of a particular family, with a part already prescribed. Indeed, parents and siblings cue us continually in their respective versions of what our actions, lines, and character ought to be. "When we enter human life," writes Bruner, "it as if we walk on stage into a play whose enactment is already in progress—a play whose somewhat open plot determines what parts we may play and toward what denouements we may be heading" (1990, p. 34). In this respect, much of our lifestory is already composed *for* us.

We shall say more on such matters under *Coauthoring*. For now, one point needs to be made. We may derive a greater portion of our sense of self-worth from the roles we play in some of the larger stories of our lives than we do from others. In the company story, we may see ourselves as indispensable, a major player at whose command everyone trembles, while at home we accept a humbler, more minor role, with much less influence or voice. In some ways, the flat role we play in the latter context is compensated for (psychologically and dramatically) by the round one we play in the former.

Narrative Environment

Within each larger story is a particular narrative environment (Bruner, 1990). Narrative environment concerns, basically, the ways people talk to each other. For example, we tend to talk to each other differently at home than we do at work or on the playing field. Narratively speaking, each is a different context, has a different climate, and elicits and allows a different way of communicating.

Narrative environment concerns the code, stated or not, as to what sorts of stories can be told and by whom, and what can or must be left *un*told. As we saw with family stories, it concerns the collection of anecdotes to which the members of a given community (variously) allude when they bring to mind what being part of that community means. As the signature stories of that community, its canon, they can in turn be catalogued according to content. In a family, for example, there will be sub-collections of *success* stories, *sickness* stories, *vacation* stories, *hard times* stories, *in-law* stories, and so on—each in each collection with its purposes for telling: to mediate values, justify habits, or meet numerous agenda at once.

Narrative environment also concerns the kinds of humor and gossip encouraged or condoned, the policies for talking with and about others. It concerns, too, the *tone* of the talk within that larger system—be it playful or pious, teasing or tense, angry or calm—and when it can shift from one to another. In general, it concerns what is permissible to talk about and what is not. Accordingly, in some larger stories, it is rigid or closed; in others, open, with members feeling free to say anything they like. Narrative environment, then, concerns not just *what* is told (or not) but *how,* in terms of concrete things like the actual vocabulary—the sayings, slang, and dialect—that is commonly used, plus the accent with which it is delivered. To participate in a certain narrative environment therefore means that we do not compose ourselves in a private language.

By learning the ways of talking—and listening—customary in these environments, we thus gain acceptance as more or less normal. We absorb a set of ways for linking events and circumstances (or "recipes for structuring experience itself") according to conventions of sense and nonsense, cause and effect—ways characterized by certain conflicts and themes, and shaped by particular genres. For example, in some families, communities, or cultures—depending on the events of their past, conditions of their present, and prospects for their future—there prevails a pessimistic, even tragic mode of talking about life. In others, a sunnier outlook reigns. To refer to what we said under plot, we learn both *what* to summarize and *how* to summarize it. We learn what is essential to tell and what is not. We learn a certain storying style.

As well, we learn whose stories possess authority, because they are deemed more tellable and valuable, are required to be listened to more, or at least are to be steered around respectfully should they remain untold. We may learn, for example, that some people are entitled to a greater share of air-time than others, who, for their part, ought to speak only when spoken to. In this way, each larger story has its own authority structure, which pressures us to compose our lives in conformity with its preferred formulas for being in the world. Such conformity is enforced rather strictly in cults, for instance, or any community committed to a particular ideology or creed. In this way, a larger story's *poetic* structure is inseparable from its *power* structure, from which voice is dominant and which is subdued.

Of the narrative environments by which we are shaped, no doubt the most potent is our family of origin. "Early in life," write Bruner and Weisser, "we learn how to talk about our lives. . . . We learn the family genre: the thematics, the stylistic requirements, the lexicon . . . procedures for offering justifications and making excuses, and the rest of it" (1991, p. 141). We might think of our own family on this point: How would we describe its narrative environment?

For instance, who did most of the talking? What did they talk about? How did they talk about it—in what genre or tone? What emphases did they place on what things; what themes did they stress; what language did they use? Was this principal narrator also the main authority figure? What topics were off limits? How were those limits enforced, and by whom? What could the others talk about? joke about? *not* talk about or joke about? Were there certain family stories we heard more frequently than others, that were the "signature stories" of the family? What were they? Who told them—as well as when and how? What were they about? What messages were embedded in them? How did they make us feel? Would our parents and siblings single out these same stories too, or think of others instead? Why? How were our own stories listened to—with impatience or respect? In general in this environment, what did we learn about both talking and listening?

If stories are not innocent, then neither is story*telling*. The way we tell our lives is inseparable from the way we live them. And the way we tell them now is rooted in the ways we *learned* to tell them as children. Our worldview, our ethics, our experience of our relationships, our gender, even our emotions—all can be traced to the way we learned to tell ourselves in the rhetorical context of family life.

Storying styles vary not only by family, of course, but also by organization (Zemke, 1990), by gender (Tannen, 1990), and, clearly, by culture (Turner and Bruner, 1986). If we were to try to explain our daily activities to our neighbors in a North American suburb using the storytelling style common to Hopi Indians—who have no tenses and thus no "normal" sense of past, present, and future (Hall, 1984)—we would soon gain the reputation for being not merely odd but probably insane. As the Gergens put it, "one cannot compose an autobiography of cultural nonsense" (1984, p. 185). "Life stories must mesh within a community of stories," echoes Bruner, "tellers and listeners must share some 'deep structure' about the nature of a 'life,' for if the rules of life-telling are altogether arbitrary, tellers and listeners will surely be alienated by a failure to grasp what the other is saying or what he thinks the other is hearing" (1987, p. 21).

Coauthoring

Implicit in the notion of narrative environment is the concept of coauthoring. As members of the same larger story, we are automatically entwined with each other's lives, not just politically but, as we are stressing, poetically too. Besides being *characters in* the stories of each other's lives, we are, intentionally or not, *coauthors of* them as well. To explain *co*authoring, we must look at authoring per se.

To return to the matter of summarizing, other people are inclined to coach us on how to talk about our lives, in terms of what to include, exclude, emphasize, ignore, and so forth. But they also coach us—it is part of the biographical imperative—in how to summarize, how to *see*, ourselves generally (Alheit, 1995). Of course, "coach" may be less accurate than "coerce," for in many cases they take on the task of storying our lives *for* us, without our consent.

From infancy to adolescence, we tend to accept others' storying of our lives as the way things are. Besides our parents, the others in question may be teachers, employers, even spouses—anyone with some degree of authority over us. With more or less bossiness, they literally "authorize" us, deliberately molding our behavior and shaping our beliefs. Often their efforts are informed by a need to "set us straight" on how we should structure our lives in terms of the larger story to which both of us adhere. Thus, the longtime believer might counsel the fresh convert, the veteran advise the rookie, or the elder instruct the initiate in "how we do things" in this religion, company, or club.

But the instruction process is not necessarily foisted on us against our will. To our parents, for example, we frequently appeal for guidance and advice, even in our adult years. Early in our lives, we implicitly give them permission (they are sure to assume it anyway) to tell us not only what to do (or *not* do) but also what to believe and how to be. In retrospect, we can be grateful for this direction, for otherwise we would have had to navigate the world on our own interpretive resources. At the time, however, it means they are constantly "after" us: *You mustn't feel that way. You mustn't think that way. You mustn't hang out with those people. Don't do that. Don't say that. Don't talk so crazy. Be a man. Be a lady. Be good.*

That is what authoring involves, and though those who are authored often give their authors a run for their money (for example, children commonly bring up their parents in the course of their parents bringing up them!), it is largely a one-way process. *Co*authoring, however, is ideally more balanced. A good example is the ordinary (if understudied) phenomenon of friendship, whether the friendships we form in adulthood or the often shorter, more intense ones of adolescence.

Without denying that family members can sometimes be friends, friends as such are people we, in a sense, intentionally enlist to make sense of our lives, especially when troubled by some problem or confused about our feelings—that is, our stories—around a relationship or event. Friends counsel us. They offer advice—respectful of our right to refuse. They help us interpret our lives in terms that are acceptable to us in some way, that blend with interpretations we have entertained in the past, or that at least do not sound too crazy—meaning, that mesh with the ways other people appear to interpret the events of *their* lives. Unless there is great inequality in our relationship, we help them do the same. Such mutual support is much of what friends are for.

Futhermore, the further back our friendships go, and the more of our lifestory our friends already know (or *think* they know), the more we may feel at home in their presence. Why? Because we trust the interpretations they provide us, or help us find for ourselves. Without regularly checking in or catching up and getting a dose of their respective versions of our lives, we may feel unsettled or unsure.

Friends authorize us. They help us make meaning—of ourselves, our relationships, our emotions, our life. But they do not merely evoke a special side of us; in a sense, they *create* it, by helping us compose our lifestory in ways we may never have before, by often very ordinary means—conversation, for instance. As philosopher Jonathan Glover puts it, "talk affects self-creation." That is, "when we talk together, I learn from your way of seeing things, which will often be different from mine. And, when I tell you about my way of seeing things, I am not just describing responses that are already complete. They may only emerge clearly as I try to express them, and as I compare them with yours. In this way, we can share in the telling of each other's inner story, and so share in creating ourselves and each other" (1988, p. 153).

The kind of telling-listening dialogue Glover describes can be relatively rare, even in therapy. In fact, in much of what we call conversation listeners hear little of what tellers say. Rather, they take their cues from what they *think* they hear (which is a summary of the teller's own summary) and, as soon as they can interrupt, strike off in a direction of their own, making the path of much chitchat a twisty one indeed. That such exchanges are commonly satisfying to tellers and listeners alike is one of the great mysteries of life. Nonetheless, Glover raises a possibility that cannot be ignored: If we could experience this quality of conversation on a regular basis, the limitations on our self-creation could be comparatively low and our sense of authorship strong. A corollary of this possibility is that the meaning we make in our lives is linked to the company we keep (Booth, 1988).

It is possible, however, that though we possess a wide range of friends, the ones we consider our best may simply be those whose version of us we particularly like—because it is most flattering, for instance, or most in harmony with our preferred version of ourselves, which knowing them keeps alive. Furthermore, something about their whole storying style resonates with our own, even if the actual *content* of their lifestory is rather foreign. On the other hand, friends with a much different version of us and a much different storying style, we may find too unsettling to be with, even though they intrigue us precisely *because* of these differences.

How friends influence our development is of course more complicated than these observations imply. But from them stem three points. First, when we switch friends, we switch versions of ourselves. Second, not just friends but anyone with whom we deal helps coauthor us to some degree (as we do them), and by the most commonplace means. Thus, little more than a warm smile or a kind word at just the right time (even from a total stranger) can give us an entirely new slant on our lives, and seed our imagination with a more self-affirming version of who we are and what we can be—a version that, in the appropriate narrative environment, can come to full fruit. Third, since coauthoring is a constant of all interaction, our lifestories are always "interknitted" (Gergen and Gergen, 1984). The texts of our lives are interwoven, never completely, of course, but enough that where our lifestory ends and another's begins can be difficult to say, as in most marriages or long-term relationships. Novel though it be, no one's life is an island.

In the next two chapters, we return to coauthoring as we consider certain practical and ethical issues surrounding the storytelling-storylistening exchange—particularly in relation to therapy and the intervention in a person's self-storying that it intentionally involves.

SETTING

The several larger stories by which we are shaped form a complex web of influences that is, in effect, the everchanging *setting* in which we tell the stories we are. A story must have a setting. We cannot compose a tale about someone doing something in an existential vacuum—unless it is a science fiction one about events unfolding inside a black hole! There must be a place where the story can *take* place.

Setting a believable setting (or set of settings, as there are often more than one) is a critical part of the storying art. It involves filling in needed details concerning color and weather and space; describing correctly the quality of light, the look of buildings and objects, the lay of the land; and simulating "just so" the requisite ambience—a hint here, an allusion there, neither too much nor too little. Appreciating how setting interacts with plot and character, genre and style, is the critic's subtle task, but it is also the social scientist's, for our *life*stories do not unfold in a vacuum either. They, too, are set somewhere in time and space. And these various settings in which we live—whether by the accident of birth, the vicissitudes of history, or conscious choice—deeply influence "the fictional side of human nature" (Hillman, 1975).

Take architecture, for instance. As Flynn puts it, writing about "Community As Story" (1991), "cultural artifacts are the setting for the story, and each monument, each building has a special meaning within the story" (p. 24). Grow up in a high-rise overlooking a freeway, a cabin in the forest, a tenement in the slums, or a mansion atop Snob Hill and the view of nature—of the world, of society—that we soak in through each setting will be unique. Or take geography. "Geography," says Australian novelist Patrick White, "is what makes us" (Hodgins, 1993, p. 77). Grow up on the prairies, and the sky and the wind live forever inside us. Grow up in the mountains and the mountains live inside us, too; their peaks and valleys, their majesty and aloofness, are always just under our skin. Grow up in the jungle, on the farm, or beside the sea and, in some unresearchable way, we are lastingly bewitched by the spell of their respective powers.

Move from one venue to another in the course of our life, and our sense of place will change accordingly, becoming more nuanced, more conflicted perhaps, but it will never disappear. As confirmation, we need only drive down the main street of our hometown after half our life has passed us by, the same town we could not wait to escape when we were eighteen and thought would afterward have no impact at all. Yet, as a flood of happy-sad memories overwhelms us with confusing nostalgia, we discover how profoundly such a setting is settled in our soul. (The place is in our story, just as our story is on some level *in* the place. We can take the child out of the hometown, that is, but not the other way around.) Economically, politically, generationally as well—if we are dragged through a depression, made redundant in a recession, or conscripted in a war, the stresses of these larger phenomena will likely leave deep marks on our philosophy of life.

It is one thing to identify the settings through which our story has moved; it is another to quantify their effects. But acknowledging their existence is a promising step. Indeed, poets and dramatists, novelists and biographers, have done so, convincingly, for years. We need only think how many authors—Faulkner, Laurence, Munro, Steinbeck, Wolfe, to name but a few—have kept returning to their roots, to mine the geography of their youth: the original settings, the early themes, the influential characters, the long unresolved conflicts that they absorbed by osmosis and, ever since, have been transforming, perhaps redeeming, into art.

This said, it is time for us who are digging our way into the mystery of the human condition from the side of social science to join those who have been hacking away from the humanities as well. Indeed, the merging of such efforts is happily evident in a number of fields already. In gerontology, for example, there is the work of Thomas Cole on *The Journey of Life* (1992), as well as the recent publication of the *Handbook on the Humanities and Aging* (Cole et al., 1992). There is also the fourth edition of the *Handbook on the Psychology of Aging* which features contributions on religion and spirituality and on narrative approaches to personality theory (Birren and Schaie, 1996). We take these as signs of an eventual rapprochement between the two cultures by whose competing claims the field of human knowledge has too long been torn.

CONCLUSION

The stories we carry around inside us are not innocent. They are bound up with our whole way of being in the world, inseparable from the relationships we enjoy, emotions we feel, and commitments we make. The story we tell is the story we *are*. Our lifestory is, effectively, our life. How we *compose* that lifestory, and thus how we form ourselves, has been our focus throughout this chapter.

Though this lifestory has been shaped by the various larger stories in which we are enmeshed—though much of its content and form has already been composed *for* us—we have in significant measure composed it for ourselves. Thus, more than we think, we possess the author-ity to *re*-compose it too. In fact, a virtual infinity of versions can be spun—and thus lives constructed—from the same body of life events. Taking authority for this construction is our focus in the chapter to come.

A postscript is in order, however, about the perspective we are proposing. One aspect of the social science enterprise that can leave many people cold is, more than the disembodied language in which its theorizing is often written, the aridity and unrootedness of its theories themselves. Not that they are without value, nor that our studies of human nature have not been advanced by means of them, but in extracting theories from real lives, perhaps we have come to exalt theories *above* lives, as if the latter were interesting and valuable only insofar as they lead to interesting and valuable theories. As we said in Chapter 1, the theory takes on a permanency it may not deserve; the finger is mistaken for the moon. In consequence, whatever we gain in analysis we may lose in understanding—in appreciating the rich uniqueness of our storied lives amid our storied worlds.

Having said this, we realize that a poetic perspective on self-creation is itself just another theory. But, it is a theory—a way of seeing—that may help put the psyche back in mainstream psychology. It may help us recover the actual feel of those dimensions of our everyday world that are supposedly the focus of *social* science. It may help us forge a more soulful, more inside-ful, science of human life.

Chapter 5

The Restorying of Our Lives

We need to reinvent ourselves continually, weaving new themes into our life narrative, remembering our past, revising our future, reauthoring the myth by which we live.

Sam Keen (1988)

INTRODUCTION

To live is to change, both outside and in. Not only do our bodies change and our circumstances, but so do our ideas, emotions, and beliefs. Mostly, this change is so gradual that we scarcely notice it, except for periodic reminders of the subtle transformations that have come with passing time. Occasionally, it is dramatic: a sudden conversion from which we emerge what seems a new person. Either way, change is the constant of our lives.

In this chapter, we look through storied lenses at the *inside* of personal change. Since who we are is a function of the stories we tell, as these change, *we* change. Passively accepted or actively aimed, this change is effectively the "restorying" of our life. Having considered the storying of our lives, we now have a sense what *re*storying involves. Thus, in what follows we do not so much add new ideas as elaborate insights already introduced.

First, we look at restorying a life as a *fact* of life, whether gradual or dramatic, natural or intentional. Next, we consider the range of ways we are moved to assume authorship of our lives and to pry ourselves loose from stories that have lived us in the past. Then, we catalogue a number of resources that can assist such restorying. Finally, we lay out the main stages of the process itself, plus the roles we can play for one another amid them, particularly story*listening*.

RESTORYING AS A FACT OF LIFE

A story is like a river: it cannot stand still. It has to go somewhere, to unfold, to flow. As it does, it becomes a *different* story. Lifestory is the same.

Given what we said about novelty in Chapter 3, the change we experience in the course of ordinary living can be compared to our experience in reading a novel. Chapter by chapter, page by page, the story steadily thickens. From its first sentence, when our commitment to reading is relatively low, when we could easily back out and put the book down, a spell is cast, an atmosphere created, and a story-line spun that sheer curiosity requires us to grab. Once we do, we are drawn deeper and deeper *into* the story. As this story-line lengthens and new events are woven into it, it takes new twists and turns. As well, new characters get introduced (thus new relationships) and new themes developed. Furthermore, new meanings can be pulled from it and pondered. There is more going on, thus more incentive for us to stay with it to see where it leads. However, though the story we thought we were getting into in the beginning has not quite disappeared, it is no longer there in the way that it was. It is the same story, yet different.

Our lifestories change in similar ways. We grow up, leave home, fall in love, start a family of our own. In turn, our children grow up, leave home, start families themselves. With more events, more people, more memories, more things to notice and tuck away, our story-world thickens. And the more it must take in, the more its boundaries stretch; it becomes steadily bigger. While the dreams of our youth are not completely eclipsed, the story we thought we were getting into as a child is thus no longer there, making all of us "exiles from our past" (Salaman, 1982, p. 55). It is the same old story, yet, daily, it is different, for "we are constantly having to revise the plot as new events are added to our lives" (Polkinghorne, 1988, p. 150). Each moment in the present provides a fresh vantage point for re-viewing the past, just as with each glance in the rear-view mirror some new contour reveals itself in the ever-receding countryside through which we drive.

All life long, we are thus involved in "continuous modifications and adjustments in [our] biographical tableau" (Berger, 1963, p. 61). In fact, this is what development is. Says developmentalist Linda Viney, it "occurs when people interpret and reinterpret their experiences of events"; its primary task is the "integration of these reinterpretations" (Botella and Feixas, 1993, p. 308). From a Sartrean perspective, the meaning of our past is thus "something that develops throughout life" (Charmé, 1984, p. 40). That is, "each act in a person's life integrates itself into a larger structure that is always developing as an organic whole" (p. 35). As we saw in considering story-time, our past is alive: ever-changing, infinitely restoryable. Though we visit its contents a thousand times, it remains a foreign country.

Such natural restorying is a fact of our life *in time*. But less gradual restorying can be a fact of life as well. Cancer strikes, an earthquake hits, a war begins, a marriage ends, and more radical restorying is forced on us. The foundations are shaken. Or there is a shift in the larger stories in which we live, and the flow of our life is diverted all at once. Whether we want to or not, we must start afresh, reworking our sense of who we are and where we are going, and what sort of world we share. Such restorying jolts us from the lulled state in which, otherwise, we might "squander our authorship" (Polster, 1987) by acquiescing to life's inevitable change, never stopping to critique its direction. Once we stop, however, it is hard to turn back. Thus, with the autobiographical imperative sounding louder within us, we elect to take charge of the restorying ourselves. Rather than react willynilly to forces that foist change upon us, we decide to craft that change ourselves, to take authority for composing our lives.

TAKING AUTHORITY FOR RESTORYING OUR LIVES

Our lifestory is the way the world *is* for us. It is what we see our world through, "the genre through which events become experiences" (Hillman, 1975, p. 146), the dynamic grid through which we make sense of our reality. Our tendency, though, is to drift along without noticing its existence (or our existence *in* it), without questioning why we live in terms of this story and not some other. What moves us, then, to take authorship of our lifestory rather than defaulting to that of others? What pushes us "to abdicate from those stories into which [we] were born and which have defined [us] and lived [us]" (Parry and Doan, 1994, p. 40)? It is the realization that the old story, however expanded by the flow of normal life, no longer gets us through. It does not work anymore. It is *dys*functional. The answers it offers fail to apply to the new questions we face.

However, the problem is not so much our history ("the facts" of our life) as the *story* in which we have put that history (Hillman, 1989). It is a familiar principle: changing how we *see* things is necessary to changing things themselves. It is not our existence that needs revision so much as our experience, not the content of our life but the form in which we have cast it in memory and imagination. For one reason or another, it does not "sufficiently represent [our] lived experience" (White and Epston, 1990, p. 14).

Of course, the fit between lifestory and life is never perfect. The tale we entertain of ourselves is always a bit off the mark, too high (or delusional) in some respects and too low (or self-deprecating) in others. To bring our self-versions more in line with our lived experience and so minimize the potential problems (personal and interpersonal) caused by the misfit between the two, some stock-taking of our storying is thus essential. The shifts in our lives that prompt it can be understood in terms of three of the elements we looked at before: plot, character, and setting.

Plot

In the last chapter, we saw plot as the the principle of *selection*, *direction*, and *coherence* that transforms raw events into story. In terms of *selection*, the need for intentional change gets sparked when we realize that events are occurring for which our old story can no longer account, because it is too simplistic or too small. Such a realization leaves us two choices: either "change the events to accommodate the story" or "change the story to accomodate the events" (Carr, 1986, p. 61).

For example, the old story is that I am healthy as a horse, have come from a long line of long livers, and will grow to a ripe, old age. This is how I have thought of myself all along. The new reality, though, is that I have cancer and only a year to live. Or, the old story is that my marriage is for keeps and my partner will be faithful till death. The reality is that the love of my life is sleeping with someone else. Or, the old story is that I am a loser, with neither talent nor brain, while the reality is that I have written four novels and am widely acclaimed for my work.

In each case, the first choice (change the events to accommodate the story) is difficult, but not impossible. Logically, yes; poetically, no—as long as we remain in denial: *It was a mistake; they mixed up the test results.* Or *Yes, they spent the night together, but nothing happened.* Or *Okay, I've accomplished a thing or two but someday they'll realize what a fraud I really am.*

The second choice (change the story to accommodate the events) involves a fundamental adjustment in our sense of who we are. Though potentially more difficult than the first, it opens the way to a new and wider lease on our life. It opens the way for us to *revise* our lifestory, to subject it to radical reformulation. Inspiring us is the realization that we need no longer be the victim of our own biography (Botella and Feixas, 1993).

In terms of *direction*, awareness of the need to make intentional change is ignited when we realize, first, the direction our life-course is taking and, second, that we do not much like it. For example, we realize that our life is "not going anywhere," or going toward a future no longer of our choosing.

Or we sense that we are moving out of one chapter and into another. Or our life-plot, *as we have composed it*, no longer charms us; it is too predictable. Or we feel we have become hostages to our own guiding myth, trapped inside it, able to do "nothing else but live out [its] plot . . . to the end" (Pearson, 1989, p. xx).

Awareness of the need to rework our lifestory is also thrust on us when our "sense of an ending" (Kermode, 1966) must suddenly change. For example, after last week's loss, our dream will never come true: the gold medal, the Oscar, or the presidency will never be ours. Or we are disillusioned when a long-held vision of how our life will turn out proves invalid—*they rejected my application; he loves me not; she's leaving for good.* The story-world we had been composing for ourselves, the life we imagined ourselves living, will no longer come to pass, and we must construct another in its place.

In terms of *coherence*, the need to make intentional change dawns on us when we realize that things are not making sense anymore, that the pieces no longer fit. Essential to everyday life, we have seen, is a feeling for the "storiedness" of our lives. This feeling, which we relate to narrative intelligence, is fundamental to our functioning in the world. Without it, we could not form dynamic impressions of each other's actions and intentions; nor see the link between our past, present, and future; nor indeed plot our life-course. Having a sense for the storiedness of our life means feeling that its details are not scattered helterskelter but entwined in one dynamic web. It means feeling that on some level event X causes or leads to event Y; that there are *reasons* things happen; that they mean something, however hard we find it to figure those meanings out.

To the extent this feeling is lacking, we experience our life not as a relatively integrated whole, but as a jumble of disconnected sensations— what Oliver Sacks calls "a Humean being" (1985, p. 30), referring to British philosopher David Hume, who saw the self as merely "a bundle of impressions." Too little of this feeling and we teeter on the brink. In the words of novelist Ursula Le Guin: "an inability to fit events together in an order that at least seems to make sense, to make the narrative connection, is a radical incompetence at being human. So seen, stupidity could be defined as a failure to make enough connections, and insanity as severe repeated error in making connections—in telling The Story of My Life" (1989, p. 43). As this feeling of disconnectedness builds, our frustrations rise—until we do what we must to "get it together."

Character

As we have seen repeatedly, our story of ourselves is tied to our stories of others, as well as to theirs of us. We live in the world only by characterizing each other continually, then relating to each other in terms of these characterizations. Frustration with these characterizations—whether ours of others, others' of us, or ours of ourselves—can also spark the need to restory.

As for our characterizations of others, we realize that we have been laboring under the wrong impression: putting them on a pedestal perhaps, or putting them down—either way, failing to appreciate how rich they really are, or how different from what we previously supposed. For example, they do or say something that seems "out of character," suddenly revealing a side of themselves invisible before, whether wild or wise, violent or kind. Of course, this side could have been there all along but was screened out because we insisted on treating them in terms of our own unfulfilled fantasies or unresolved past; that is, we saw *their* lifestory through ours. Equally, they could be genuinely changing, intentionally restorying. Either way, we realize we have been "storyotyping" them unfairly, constructing a working image of them based on inadequate information. Formerly flat in our perception, they thus begin to round out, to come alive. And as they change in our imagination, we must change in our own. Because they are co-actors in *our* lifestory, a change in their role requires adjustment in ours.

As for others' characterizations of us, the impetus to restory comes with the realization that one or other of the people in our lives—a parent, spouse, or friend—is not a *co*author *with* us so much as an author *over* us, that they are constantly (if subtly) instructing us what to do and think and feel. Instead of seeing us as a responsible agent capable of designing our own life, or an equal partner acceptable as we are, they view us as someone who can be *told* who we are, can be pushed into *their* image of who we ought to be. This realization, which often dawns in adolescence, sparks our spirit of independence, piques the autobiographical imperative, and unleashes the desire to claim our own authorship. If their authority has been sufficiently invasive, however, we may keep this spirit suppressed, and so suffer lifelong doubt about our capacity to create an identity for ourselves.

Or it may work the other way around: Someone new comes along who refuses to tell us who we should be, who subverts the authority we otherwise accord them. Instead, they insist on loving us as we are, or on believing in us when we are unable to believe in ourselves. In this way, they sow the seeds of a more liberating version of our life, and coax from us the courage to compose it on our own terms.

In addition, when certain people who have been close to us fall ill, walk out, or pass on, they take with them the version of us, positive or negative, that they regularly reinforced, the side they habitually evoked. Depending how deeply we had internalized this version as who we are, their departure *de*-stories us, at least temporarily. After a period of disorientation, we may find we relish the opportunity with which we are now presented: to re-characterize as someone new.

As for our characterizations of ourselves, realization of the need to restory can come with no more exotic a development than becoming bored with the role we have been assigned in the drama of the family, the marriage, or the company. We tire of spouting the usual lines that everyone has come to expect of us; they no longer suit our emerging sense of ourselves. We weary of the same scenarios, the same tug-of-war, the same irritatingly crude ways of being perceived by our co-actors (and perhaps by ourselves) as villain or victim, and so on. We sicken of being treated storyotypically, and of living the lie that others believe we are. Thus, in some stubborn part of ourselves we decide to break free of their perceptions and stop caring what they think.

Also, we may feel the need to restory to the degree that we weary of the underlying myth by which we have understood ourselves to date, perhaps after a particular incident has given us a glimpse of how, generally, we move through the world. As a result, we stop believing the legend we have made of our lives. We find it limiting. Little by little, we elect to break free of it and invent ourselves afresh—to re-genre-ate, perhaps: from a *woe-is-me* (or tragic) orientation to a more proactive, adventurous one. For example, Carol Pearson—who invites us to make "explicit the myths that govern our lives" (1989, p. xx)—challenges women to push past the martyr archetype that has traditionally been held out to them as the only role worth living. Similarly, she dares men to critique the warrior archetype to which they are commonly conditioned and in which so many stay stuck.

Another way we can be prompted to change our self-characterization is by others' reactions to an achievement that—to them, to us—seems out of character. It constitutes a unique outcome that fails to fit with the dominant story by which we identified ourselves before (White and Epston, 1990). (Sometimes, we do or say things that surprise not only others but also ourselves!) If the feedback we receive is steady and strong, it amounts to new information that must be incorporated into our sense of our potential.

It helps us catch a vision of another whole side of ourselves, another sub-personality, with its own plot line that begs to be lived.

However, such feedback usurps not just the cherished view we have held of our future but the perception we have had of our past. In light of recent accomplishments, there may be things in our past we can now celebrate, of which we were previously ashamed. When the press applauds our first novel, for example, we reevaluate the years of poverty we poured into writing: not as the mark of the dreamer we were dismissed so long for being, but of a great artist who was tried in the creative fire until his time could eventually come.

Setting

Last chapter, we spoke of the *setting* of our lifestory as an interlocking of larger stories that constitute our narrative home—stories we tend to see (and trust) not as "just stories" but as the way things *are*. For not only are we inside of them, but they are inside of *us*. The traces of their texts deeply penetrate our lives, making where we end and they begin impossible to say. Thus, when they change, so must we. In essence, our old story no longer works in the new setting.

A simple example is a geographical one: moving from X to Y as a child. A new village or neighborhood—each with its own history, myth, and story—represents a new *con*text in which to weave the text of our lives and be knit with those of others. Through our pores, we absorb new conflicts, new themes, new plot lines, new characters. Storywise, we are thrown into a whole different world. If it is too unfamiliar, however, we are (literally) unsettled. Deep inside ourselves, albeit within the protective story-world of our immediate family, we must rework our sense of who we are. Moving from a quiet rural world to a noisy urban one, we find its authority and morality, its whole narrative environment, disturbingly different—more complex or more free—than that from which we came.

Another example is being shifted from the story-world of one household to that of another because our parents divorce and we must move into a new or blended family. For a while, the actors in the drama of this arrangement will be following a script on which the ink is still wet. No one knows where the new plot is likely to go, nor each player's lines and roles. Accordingly, our "character" must change—as must the entire life-trajectory we had previously imagined. The same applies not just in childhood or adolescence, of course, but in adulthood too—when we go from one intimate relationship to another, and must accommodate ourselves to a new *couple* story.

But among the larger stories of our lives are also the company in which we work, the creed to which we subscribe, and the culture and gender to which, by birth, we belong. If one of these suffers a significant shift—the firm goes bankrupt, the city is bombed, the country splits apart—then these large-scale events will effect a change in the conditions (natural, political, economic) in which our personal, couple, and family stories unfold, so dominating our day-to-day lives that our old ways of composing ourselves no longer fit. Where restorying those conditions is out of the question because out of our control, restorying ourselves is our only resort. Where it is not, however, we may discover we can make a difference, that the personal and political converge, that in restorying ourselves we force reform on the systems that otherwise limit our lives.

This suggests that change is not always initiated from the side of the larger stories themselves, but, often, from our side, living *within* them. Such change is prompted when a given larger story, though unfolding fine as it is, weighs upon us as "the same old story." We see it differently than we did; where once it was home, now it is a strange land, or a prison. Thus, we find ourselves impatient to break out, as did Tom Baxter, the hero of a Woody Allen movie called *The Purple Rose of Cairo*, who walked off the screen and out of his role. It can be for no more philosophical a frustration than this, in fact, that many of us eventually leave home, end a marriage, or quit a job.

Sometimes, the frustration that drives us to exit a larger story—to extricate ourselves from its *con*text—has more passion. We realize that it not only embraces our personal story but actively oppresses it, denies it, silences it. There is a battle of stories within us: its against ours. Our disenchantment with its whole ethos may thus increase to where we opt out of it altogether and into another from which it is fundamentally different— as communism is from capitalism, or Judaism from atheism. Or, to cite a more individual example: as someone adopted as a child, we may opt to track down our parents and return to our roots.

RESOURCES FOR RESTORYING

When we move from restorying continuously to restorying consciously—to actively authoring our lives—a number of resources are ready to help us. In terms of what they offer and how they function, these resources are either formal or informal. In the formal category are the official, more or less formulaic programs we are presented in education, religion, and therapy. In the informal group are the freer, subtler influences we encounter in art, other people, and ourselves. We now consider each of these in turn, ending with an approach to restorying—guided autobiography—that incorporates several resources at once.

Education

From nursery school to graduate school, formal education is a system for storying the world, where storying is a synonym for making meaning. As such, any program, institution, or course sits on a continuum between two extremes.

At one end, meaning is made *for* us. It is packaged in advance, then force-fed to us to regurgitate on the final exam. Accordingly, education is the *transmission* of knowledge—about our universe, our society, ourselves—from experts through teachers to students. At the other end, we are supplied with basic concepts and information, plus a supportive and stimulating environment, then encouraged to make meaning on our own—in the process often *re*making ourselves and our world. Accordingly, education is a matter of *transformation*. In the former model, we are passive receivers of knowledge; in the latter, active creators.

Traditionally, education has been equated with the former model—the conduit model (Ortony, 1979)—and thus with regulation and regimentation. We are told what to believe, instructed in what is true, and informed about who we are: consumers in economics class, statistics in sociology, a mass of molecules in science. As students in a given educational program—indoctrinated in certain principles, imbued with certain theories, and schooled in certain methods—we are literally discipline-d into a particular way of interpreting both our world and ourselves. To go to school is therefore to submit to having our lives storied *for* us.

This model of education may seem overly dismal, for knowledge can also set us free. This includes knowledge about ourselves, such as the knowledge we acquire in psychology class that we are not "slow" like we have always been labeled but that our learning style merely requires more time to process our thoughts, which may in fact be more solid than those of our quick-thinking peers. In general, the love of learning for learning's sake, which learning such things unleashes, can liberate our soul. As it does, we find no limit to what we can know—that the world is our classroom, that the most innocuous incident or most ordinary day is a text from which some lesson can be gleaned. We find sermons in stones and books in running brooks. Our classroom, then, can also be ourselves.

This latter model of education is always struggling to break through the former, more authoritarian approach. In it, we are empowered to be critical thinkers, to consult our own experience, and out of that experience to compose a story of ourselves and a vision of our world that derives its authority from within, not without. Such an approach to education—which one scholar calls "biographical learning" (Alheit, 1995)—runs through the feminist movement, the popular education movement, and much of the movement known as adult education. Put crudely, its motto is to "tell *our* story, our *whole* story, and *nothing but* our story." Synonymous with such an approach is what Jack Mezirow calls "transformative learning," at the core of which is "learning how we are caught in our own history and are repeating it" (1978, p. 101). Wilhelm Mader sees the facilitation of such learning as central. Indeed, even though "very often [it] happens under the surface of the learning process . . . there is no educational material, no subject matter, that would not be able to trigger any biographical self-reflection at all" (1995, p. 245).

In a provocative book called *Narrative Schooling*, Richard Hopkins (1994) urges educators to conceive even conventional (K–12) institutions "as places where students construct and share their stories" (pp. 126, 132), and to see students, like all of us, as motivated by a fundamental "narrative impulse" (p. 3)—what we are calling the autobiographical imperative. With these conceptions informing them, he says, teachers will see their task as supporting students in "a narrative exercise, helping them to construct and tell their stories in continuous narrative portfolios, using the materials of the world (including the traditional academic subjects) to understand the past, manage the present, and plan the future" (p. 8). Rather than subjects having priority over students, then, subject matter only "comes to life when it is associated with the actual narrative structures of real people living (and planning) their lives" (p. 147). In a school based on the narrative root metaphor, students work a great deal in groups, where the focus is on making meaning by conscious coauthoring: "each group member narrates a sense of his or her past life, present life, and anticipated future among other people—a reflective and constructive process, an intersubjective exercise in the formation of self" (p. 142).

Religion

More obvious than education as a resource for restorying is religion. As we saw last chapter, what any religion offers is "a great master narrative" (Cupitt, 1991) that, quite unabashedly, purports to answer our questions about where the world has come from and where it is going. As well, it pronounces on the nature of human nature, on the meaning of life, on what to do (or not do) between birth and death, and indeed on who we *are*, whether *sinner* or *child of God*. Such a narrative is a myth in the classic sense, not something automatically unscientific or untrue, and not an illusion as Freud would say, but a mythos: a guiding plot by which the world is rendered coherent to us, so we can live with meaning and hope. So understood, it is not only religion in the narrow sense that offers myths by which to live, but in the broad sense too: any creed, philosophy, or ideology that expounds an authoritative story for us to adhere to "religiously" in living and telling our own.

Naturally, advocates and authorities for each religion (or ideology) are unlikely to see themselves as promoting just a story. On the contrary, the interpretation of things that lies at the heart of their faith can be believed so fiercely that they consider it true—not an interpretation, but reality, solid and sure: nailed down with doctrine, enshrined in symbol, and confirmed by holy writ. In turn, the story they revere is inseparable from the world they experience and the life they lead. Thus, we can never understand the ethics or theology of a given tradition without knowing the story at its base.

As with education, so with religion: from one faith to another, the stories in which followers are indoctrinated show significant differences, ones that have had centuries to develop. The vision of the world we are taught in Christianity can be worlds removed from what we learn in Shinto or Zen, in animism or Islam. Also, any tradition or denomination, congregation or sect, will tend toward one of two extremes in enforcing conformity of life and thought. In fundamentalist circles, the prescribed story (both of the world and of us) is tightly told and strictly edited; alternative versions are shunned. In liberal circles, it is more fluid, more open; we are invited to read into it what meanings we need or can; a wider range of interpretations is tolerated. Either way, when we look to (or through) a formal religious system, it is to a particular program for restorying that we shall be enjoined to convert. To the degree that it helps us make sense of our lifestory material, it will comfort us with the feeling of having found a narrative home in which to compose our lives in peace. If sufficiently euphoric, this feeling will signal rebirth.

However, many of us become frustrated with the rigidity of the life prescribed by the religion into which we are born. Not just because we find its moral code naive or unrelated to the real world but because we can no longer subscribe to the story it would have us believe—about the cosmos, about history, about ourselves. Furthermore, our suspicion of all such "master narratives" may intensify with our awareness of how deep can be the conflict—the battle of stories—between entire traditions, whether the case be Northern Ireland or the Middle East. It may be fueled as well by our sense that the authority of *any* religion is undermined by science.

However, the authority of science is itself increasingly questioned. Postmodern critiques of the scientific method see it as, fundamentally, a "storying" enterprise (Gergen and Gergen, 1986; Cupitt, 1991). Scientists traffic less in facts than in interpretations, in versions of natural events. Like religion, science is a spinner of tales. Each theory it proposes to account for a given phenomenon is ultimately a *story,* about what has happened and why, and what might happen next.

With such skepticism about the ability of both science and religion to lead us to truth, there is a deep desire within many of us, then, for a small "s" spirituality in which we can discover and savor our own unique story, listen deeply to the stories of others, and construct collective stories whose authority does not descend from on high but emerges from within. As put by one theologian, if "we are all asking, 'what stories can we live by,'" then "one way to begin to answer that question is to start telling our own stories" (Keen, 1993, p. 30). Though it is not our purpose to outline it here, such a spirituality could be profoundly freeing. In it, whatever structure, direction, and revelation we seek would come from inside us, and among us. A different coauthoring would prevail than the coercive kind common in sectarian circles, where open-ended conversation (such as we talked about in the last chapter) is discouraged in favor of a controlled exchange in which all self-telling is conducted in line with official doctrine concerning what counts as a spiritual life. But because such spirituality could be freeing, it might also be frightening, opening us to a "metaphysical agoraphobia" brought on by "one of the most terrifying ideas the mind can have," which is "that this or any other conversion is not necessarily final, that one could be reconverted and re-reconverted" (Berger, 1963, p. 63).

Such continual conversion is integral to the vision of psychologist James Fowler in *Stages of Faith* (1981). Fowler, who uses faith as a verb more than a noun, sees it as a "human universal" that "functions so as to screen off the abyss of mystery that surrounds us." Faith "helps us form a dependable 'life space,' an ultimate environment" (pp. xii–xiii), that gives us hope, a reason for being. Moreover in his view, it grows in predictable stages. If we accept the premise of Gregory Bateson that "we select and edit the reality we see to conform to our beliefs about what sort of world we live in" (Engel, 1972, p. vii), then in Fowler's framework movement from one stage to another is inevitable as we continually revise our versions of the stories we are.

Therapy

As resources for restorying, education offers us food for thought—or food for the mind—while religion offers food for the spirit. What therapy promises is food for the soul, which in Greek is *psyche*, from which we get psych-ology. *Therapy* we can take in a broad sense as including not only psychoanalysis and psychotherapy but also social work, counseling, spiritual direction, family therapy, indeed any process in which one person offers another an organized perspective on his life: how best to understand it and change it.

Of course, the transformative influences of all three—education, religion, and therapy—are commonly connected, in at least two ways. First, underlying any therapeutic perspective is an implicit theory of learning. (In a sense, all therapy is educational, and all education therapeutic.) Plus, there will be biases at work that are arguably theological in origin—as is the case with certain schools of existentialist or humanistic psychology. Second, in choosing to change our lives, we often elect to feed mind, spirit, and soul all at once. Thus, we may reach out in numerous directions simultaneously: going back to school, exploring spirituality, and visiting a counselor. Our point is simply that when people seek deliberately to restory their lives, there are many ways to go about it. Formal therapy is ever only one. It may not even be the most effective (at least for certain individuals), despite the favored status it has acquired in the Western world. However, the demise of the modernist mentality is raising questions about therapy's methods and merits.

We shall return to this point later. For now, as in education and religion, so in therapy. The array of resources into which we can tap is equally broad. For the restructuring of our own lives—or "the restorying of experience" (White and Epston, 1990)—each therapeutic school prescribes a set of story lines that are more or less explicitly articulated and rigidly interpreted. Thus, an orthodox Freudian analyst guides the retelling or reauthoring of our lifestory in accordance with the Oedipal myth (Schafer, 1992), while a diehard Jungian or Adlerian employs another myth instead. Different again is the approach of the eclectic, client-centered therapist who draws on a variety of theoretical perspectives and attempts to listen to our story on its own terms before recommending, broker-like, a perspective from which we might draw.

In the next chapter, we will return to this issue of the therapeutic master story that guides a given telling-listening exchange, for it has important ethical implications, as does the issue of how long a therapist and client actually work together. Where their relationship spans months or years, the therapist, as keeper of the patient's old lifestory and host of the new one being created, possesses a disturbing degree of authority, in which the interpretative work their analysis involves "may determine the past more clearly than even the past itself" (Spence, 1982, p. 94). For now, we want merely to underline what became obvious in Chapter 1 in surveying those using the story metaphor to generate working concepts for the therapeutic process—concepts like coauthoring, emplotment, and narrative truth. As such terms take their place in the lexicon of social science, they will show that we are shifting from a predominantly psychodynamic model of human nature to a more thera*poetic* one.

Art

What art "is" is probably a mystery. What it does, we could say, is present us a transforming vision of our surroundings and ourselves. It offers issues to consider, questions to ponder, and, if we are open, insights by which to be edified and enriched. In the case of music or the visual arts, it manages this by acting on our emotions rather directly. With the narrative arts (plays or novels, for instance), the process is more roundabout, insofar as they appeal to our emotions by means of a story. However, to the degree, or for the duration, that we identify with this story, it becomes *our* story. Through it, we see ourselves and make sense of our world.

As in education, religion, and therapy, we have the same range of options. Two broad types of stories tend to get told: the conventional, close-ended, formulaic type that we find in romance novels action-thriller films, and weekly TV dramas, and the inventive, open-ended type that are "novel" in that they offer us something original in both content and form. As such, they represent what the philosopher Collingwood calls "art properly so-called."

In the former, meaning is made *for* us, leaving us little to do on our own. The plot lines are tight, conflicts cliché, themes familiar, characters stock. The morality is trite, the genre clear, and the final effect invariably satisfying (even addicting), if short-lived. There are also limited ways to get from a beginning to an end. Night after night, these ways are paraded before us, in sitcoms and soaps, mysteries and sports. By such stories we may be titillated and entertained, and occasionally informed, but rarely *trans*formed. If they are the staples of our imaginative diet, then our lifestory may be stunted indeed (Booth, 1988).

In the latter option, the realm of literature as such, the very form of story is constantly tested. Writers endeavor to write narratives that break from "the same old story"; that convey a question or voice a wisdom that the world would otherwise not know. They attempt to transfuse to *our* experience some aspect of their own: to connect directly with our inner world, to transform it in novel ways. To do this, they strive to lay out plot lines that do not lead us down the usual paths, to develop themes and devise conflicts that can be complex to follow (as in everyday life!), and to make reading a challenge that stretches both mind and soul. They draw out nuances of thought and feeling, and articulate ambiguities in behavior, that social science cannot (which, by method if not intention, is an outside-in endeavor, not inside-out, like art). Moreover, they create characters that are round and alive, whose illuminations and transformations provide guidance for our own lives and hope in our struggles to change them for the better. Thus, literature is "a life support system" (Gold, 1990, p. 24).

In addition, such writers push us to play with "possible worlds" (J. Bruner, 1986) long after we learn technically, how, their stories end. Whatever meaning they may intend is not announced. We must ponder it, discuss it, and, ultimately, make it ourselves. As languaged texts in which "every word is ambiguous in and of itself," these stories "have no inherent and stable meanings" anyway (McAdams, 1994, p. 781). Their meanings will always be many. Thus, literature "properly so-called" has an open-ended, dialogical quality, one that expands our "literary competence" (Spence, 1982) and tests our narrative intelligence.

Literature, writes Sven Birkerts, "remains the unexcelled means of interior exploration and connection-making" (1994, p. 197). It possesses an inherently "emancipatory potential" (Greene, 1990). Something happens when we read. Because of certain stories we become a different person. Deep reading of them dis-illusions us, loosens us from our usual interpretations and expectations amid everyday life, and opens us to transformative truths. In this way, the entire body of literature is "a human apocalypse, man's revelation to man" (Frye, 1963, p. 44), with the power to educate our imagination and enrich our experiencing of the world. Also, like the story of a religion or creed, it gives us confidence (grounded or not) in the world's essential coherence, and so "keep[s] alive the dangerous and exhilarating idea" that our life is ultimately going somewhere, that it "is not a sequence of lived moments, but a destiny" (Birkerts, 1994, p. 83). So viewed, a "good" story gives us both insight and hope.

Other People

The idea of other people as resources for restorying connects to the concept of coauthoring. As we have seen, we are continually telling one another how to act, how to make sense of events, how to interpret our world. *You mustn't think like that*; *stop that*; *your problem is that . . .* : with such phrases or their nonverbal equivalents we are forever patting each other into shape. We seldom stop to realize, however, how much our lives are thus authored *for* us; how powerfully our views and values, beliefs and behaviors, are constructed by our relationships. As soon as we are born, people start telling us who we are, sometimes assuming an authority *over* us that is decidedly unhealthy—the extreme being a cult leader who brainwashes us with his or her warped worldview in order to exploit our energies and gifts. To move from "squandering our authorship" to more actively composing our lives means, for one thing, then, picking more carefully the company we keep (Booth, 1988) and the people from whom we learn.

That we can "learn" from other people, few would deny. Much in life we can find hard to figure out. To maneuver it safely, we soon discover that we need all the insight we can get. One way to get it is in the stories of others: their relationships, their successes and failures, their struggles and mistakes. In everyone's story is a lesson to be learned. Indeed, some stories can instruct us so powerfully that we say (as we might of a novel or character therein) they "changed my life!" They inspire us by their example, by their courage, by awakening our capacity for learning or love. We can call this biographical learning; however, it is far from clear what such learning involves, nor shall we come to any conclusions concerning it here. But it bears examination in connection with restorying our lives. Accordingly, we propose that there are three types of people from whose lives—or lifestories—we commonly learn: living people, dead people, and fictional people.

Learning from the lifestories of fictional people seems simple enough. As we have hinted throughout, art affects life—by imitating it, illuminating it, investigating it, and so on—even if the mechanics of its effects are not our focus here. Suffice it to say, few of us have not been moved, not felt edified or affirmed, by our encounter with someone brought to life only by words on a page or acts on a stage. What the words and acts mediate, of course, is only that person *as constructed* by an author-narrator, or director-actor. However, as we complete the aesthetic equation, we in turn *re*-construct them by reaching into our repertoire of *lived* experience, which resonates with their *virtual* experience. Vicariously, we learn from their situations and struggles. This means that, ultimately, we are learning from ourselves, that the lifestory of the fictional character merely focuses insights we incipiently possess about our own. Says Birkerts: "I read books to read myself" (1994, p. 102).

The idea of learning from the lifestories of dead people—whether cultural heroes, religious saints, or family ancestors—presents a logical problem, the same as confronts the historian: how to access the past in the present. Yet this dilemma seldom detains us. Despite the fact that dead people are by definition dead, we persist in the belief that we can still learn from their example. Again, it is not clear how such learning happens. But one thing *is* clear: it will be prompted by reading some *text* about their actions, achievements, or thoughts, whether that text be inscribed on our own memory, written down in history books, biographies, and *auto*biographies, or passed on orally from others (though each medium will textualize them differently). Depending on how long they have been dead, how close they have been to us geographically and relationally, and through whose memories and agendas their lives are filtered, our access to their lifestories will be more or less clear—or opaque.

The lifestories of living people as resources for restorying are different from those of dead people. For one thing, they are far less fixed aesthetically; they lack the finality and the illusion of clarity that death, like literature, confers on any life. For that reason, they are harder to "read"—some more so than others, their life-texts intrinsically more conflicted, more layered or "deep." Put another way, living people keep changing on us, as do our perceptions of them and relationships with them. Thus, reading the texts of their lives is a continual process—not least because our own (through which we read) keep changing as well, as in lengthening, thickening, becoming more complex. When two lifestories become particularly interknit, as they do in any close, coauthoring relationship, this reading can go both ways—as *co*-reading—with the increased potential for learning that this will entail (insofar as two texts are more textured than one). Indeed, this is part of what pulls us to another person in the first place: the allure of their lifestory. Although largely a mystery to us at the outset, we sense something in it—something to be learned, something intriguing (because untold?)—and so, detective-like, we want to read on.

As with education, religion, therapy, and art, so with other people, living or dead. Some provide neatly packaged models of "the art of living," which in time get immortalized and legendized as examples to follow. But there can be a cardboard quality to the caricature, however holy, into which they are turned that makes the texts of their lives rather *closed* books. The lives of others present themselves more openly, less rigidly. They are *open* books. We can take from them such lessons, such meanings, as suit us—and there will always be more should we read them again. The more we get to know them, the more there is to learn.

Ourselves

Despite what we have said about the links between learning from others and learning from ourselves, many of us are uncomfortable seeing ourselves as resources for restorying. Life under the modern worldview has drummed into us that we are incapable of running our own lives, that we must look beyond ourselves for help. Hence our deference to "experts," who stand ready, we believe, to fix our every failing. Where we are all questions, they are all answers; where we are all problems, they are all solutions. In contrast to the chaos and confusion that plague our lives, they point to sanity and order. This book, however, reflects the *post*-modern view that experts are not as expert as they seem. Indeed, putting our trust in them too much has, in too many ways, led our planet to the brink.

As we have discussed, the authority of education, science, or religion lies not in any direct access it affords us to "the truth" but in the story it tells *about* the truth, a story we have the option to read, evaluate, and accept—or not. Once we accept that every theory and doctrine is merely a story about what is real, whose meaning for us is fundamentally story-meaning, not fact-meaning, then we can turn to our own *life*story with fresh respect. We can begin to see that the text of our lives is potentially as instructive as any other, however scholarly or objective it is touted to be. And as enticing too (though modern psychology has worked hard to take the *mystery* out of "my story"). Indeed, we can begin to appreciate how it is in effect a *sacred* text (Charmé, 1984), and "reading" it analagous to savoring a great novel. But such reading is not an aesthetic luxury; it is an existential need. It is the root of our ability to "know" anything at all. In the stirring words of adult educator Michael Brady,

Is this not our destiny as human beings: to learn, to grow, to come to know ourselves and the meanings of our life in the deepest, richest, most textured way possible? If we do not know the self, what can we know? If we cannot learn from reflection upon our own lived experiences, from what can we learn? (1990, p. 51)

The approach we advocate here liberates experts from the burden of our perception of them as possessing the answers. It accords them a humbler, more human role in relation to us, not with authority *over* us but as coauthors *with* us—"biographical coaches" (Alheit, 1995)—as we plot a course through the complexities of our life that reveals itself from within rather than from without. As psychoanalyst Karen Horney reminds us, "life itself remains a very effective therapist" (Kennedy, 1976, p. 124). Therapists—analysts, social workers, educators, confessors—are never the only agents of deep personal change, nor the processes of formal counseling the only avenue to achieving it. As we are seeing, such change can occur by many means and be supported by several resources. Together, they constitute a dynamic context within which we can reweave the texts of our lives. Before we look at the stages of restorying and thus of accessing the insight that resides within us, we want to consider a strategy in which a number of these resources converge.

Guided Autobiography

Guided autobiography (Birren and Birren, 1996; Birren and Deutchman, 1991) is an approach to restorying created some twenty years ago by gerontologist James Birren. Since then, it has come to be used throughout Canada, the United States, and Europe by a broad range of researchers, practitioners, and educators—at both the graduate and undergraduate levels. Wilhelm Mader (1995) utilizes it with graduate students of adult education in Germany, for example, while Gary Kenyon has shared it with doctoral students and faculty in Sweden and, for over six years, in Canada, with undergraduates in gerontology. In addition, it lends itself well to a workshop format and has tremendous potential for community development, particularly among older persons, by minimizing their sense of isolation and facilitating their involvement and reengagement.

Guided autobiography is best described as an educational, existential, even spiritual form of restorying. While it has therapeutic value, however, it is not therapy per se, a distinction we shall return to in the next chapter. Rather, it involves storylistening and storytelling in a nonjudgmental atmosphere of mutual respect, with no other explicit agenda, no "master narrative," in mind. It employs a combination of elements, among which Mader (1995) identifies five: the element of *themes*, the *written* element, the element of *personal reflection*, the element of *social communication*, and the *metaphorical* element.

Each guided autobiography session begins with a group activity in which we might discuss a particular theory of human development or examine different aspects of the story metaphor. In the second part of the session, we are introduced to a selected *theme* for the day by means of "sensitizing questions" (Birren and Deutchman, 1991) intended to get us thinking about a particular part of our lifestories. However, we are encouraged to address this theme in our own unique way, and to use poetry, literature, and *metaphors* as much as we wish.

In guided autobiography, a set of core themes are stressed because they reflect broad life—or existential—issues, and because considering them helps us access the full content of our lifestory. Exploring one, for example, entails finding a metaphor to characterize our life as a whole, whether a branching tree, a flowing river, or some other image. Other themes include the story of significant others in our life, our sexual story, our view of death and dying, and our dreams and aspirations. Still others include our story of money and stress, of spirituality and meaning. As Mader notes, these are all basic storytelling themes since "nobody can escape the necessity of developing a biographically useful relationship to death, body, money, aging, etc." (1995, p. 251). Finally, depending on the make-up of the group, particular themes may be designed in advance to reflect specific interests, such as our story of music and art or significant classroom experiences of retired teachers. The key is that these themes be flexible and reflect the interests and backgrounds represented in the group. In this respect, even a core theme will sometimes be omitted from a course, and we are always free to decide *not* to address a particular theme if it causes us discomfort.

Having been introduced to the theme for a particular session, we spend the remainder of the time, or the period until the next session, in *personal reflection* on that theme. As part of this process, we are asked to write a maximum of two pages on how that theme relates to our life. This *written* part of our story forms the basis of what is then *socially communicated*— that is, shared—in small groups during the following session. These groups normally consist of five to eight persons. The leader of each group has only two roles, both noninvasive: to keep time and thus allow all of us an opportunity to express our story, and to prevent any judgmental remarks or interpretations from damaging the open-ended, purely story*listening* nature of the process.

As for the appropriate attitude or behavior in a guided autobiography group, Kenyon's motto is that "if you have nothing good to say to someone, don't say anything at all." However, it is sometimes difficult for professional "agents of restorying" to follow such advice—in particular, to leave their hats at the door and become simply another member with a story to share. As we have said before, metaphors and stories sometimes develop their own immune system, as a result of professional training and the prolonged use of a particular storyotype. However, there is no special training required to lead a guided autobiography class, save that we have experienced the process ourselves beforehand, a point with ethical implications we will take up in the next chapter.

A common outcome of guided autobiography is that it creates an effective narrative environment for people to restory their lives together—that is, for coauthoring. Its explicitly nonfocused agenda allows them rather quickly—even if strangers at the outset—to become trusted friends. In fact, some remain friends long after the course is complete. At the very least, if the basic rule is respected of listening without judging, the almost unanimous outcome is that everyone has a positive experience of sharing their stories. More often than not, however, much *radical* restorying occurs, some examples of which we discuss in the next chapter. As a result, people report finding significant new meaning in their lives.

To conclude, an interesting question to ask of the guided autobiography approach is why it generally works so well. How, for example, does it compare with other resources such as therapy and self-help, and what is the role played in it by different "media"—namely, as we will discuss shortly, the verbal versus the written, or telling our story to ourselves versus telling it to another? Compelling as these questions are, we must now look in more detail at the restorying process itself.

THE STAGES OF RESTORYING

In the last chapter we identified different points of view from which a story can be told—that of author, narrator, protagonist, or reader. From a different point of view the story becomes a different story. If we add to this the range of rhetorical strategies at our disposal in terms of time, tone, vocabulary, and voice, then the number of stories we can extract from a given set of events is virtually limitless. There is never just one tale to tell. The same holds true in the realm of *life*story. "Anyone," say Bruner and Weisser, "can reel off multiple autobiographies of his own life" (1991, p. 135). Or as Charmé puts it, "Since there is no one 'true' description of the past, there is no one 'true text' " (1984, p. 52).

Because there is no one "true text," there is a glorious open-endedness to being who we are. This is the journey-like, adventurous quality to our lives, since our identity is malleable. Nothing is settled, neither our past, present, nor certainly our future. All is amenable to interpretation. Quips one pundit, "it's never too late to have a happy childhood." Nor, we could add, is it ever too early to have a fulfilling old age. Within reason, we can (in principle) tell, and live, whatever story we choose. Realizing this can either overwhelm us with agoraphobia at the unbounded nature of our being, or make us celebrate the possibilities it presents.

Either way, embarking on intentionally restorying our lives is a daunting endeavor. Opening the lid and peering into all this possibility can feel like staring into the abyss—in this case, a full abyss. As former UN Secretary-General Dag Hammerskjöld once admitted, "the longest journey is the journey inward." Much courage is required to enter what we fairly fear may be "the dark night of the soul." As a result, the urge to squander our authorship can become as great as our fear. Indeed, we can grow wonderfully inventive at distracting ourselves, by flicking channels, pouring another drink, consulting another expert—anything to avoid the potential misery of becoming lost in the maze of our inner world. To *e*-scape, not *in*-scape, becomes our driving desire.

Without underestimating the complexity or length of the restorying process, we can identify three overlapping, spirally-related stages: telling, reading, and retelling. Arbitrary labels, to be sure, they point to three phases of the creative process familiar to any student of English composition: writing, editing, and revising. First, we get down our ideas; next, we edit our efforts; and, finally, we rewrite, producing draft after draft until we get it right (or get blue in the face!). Applying these phases to composing the text of our lives may seem a simple-minded, language-centered depiction of the complex process of personal change. As we hope to show, however, it has its place.

Telling

Once we are willing to make the perceptual turn and look at our life *as a story*, we realize that we are telling ourselves continually. Each time we talk, we talk eventually about ourselves—our feelings, relationships, fears. We are involved in autobiographical activity all the time. *Why* we talk, however, is another story. There can be several reasons. We may talk to claim our space: to stake out a certain psychic territory as ours and not others'. But we may talk to *connect* with others, too—to influence them, inform them, get close to them. We may also talk to better understand our own thoughts—that is, to process our lives, to sort through the significance of the events and people that make them up.

The self-telling we are talking about here is not discontinuous with the type we do all the time, especially the latter—telling to sort ourselves out. Yet it is different, because more focused and profound. We engage in it with greater awareness of both what we are telling and how, with a stronger desire to get to the bottom of our lives. In other words, much everyday self-telling is functional in nature—*Pass the salt; I've got a headache; I'd like wine with my meal*—and limited in length. The unspoken stipulation in most interaction is to leave our *real* selves untold, to keep the better portion of ourselves to ourselves, and to edit ruthlessly what we do not, so we can all "get on with things" and "get along." This is true when we are on the job or out in public. But even among family and friends, we encounter countless restrictions against "going too deep" or "getting too personal," restrictions we may internalize to where we not only lose touch with our own depth but deem it weakness to be concerned with the loss. Either that, or we become embarrassingly chatty, blurting out all sorts of bits about ourselves at the least hint our listener is interested, oblivious to the signs that they are merely indulging us while waiting to embark on a monologue of their own, or excuse themselves and leave. Some of us talk too much, in other words, and our talking goes round and round in circles—the same old story again and again.

We pay a price, though, for bottling our lives inside. It leads to frustration, much of which we are conditioned to forbid ourselves to feel. That is, we accept a certain silence about ourselves as just the way things are. Indeed, many *men* have not only accepted the way of silence but elevated it to a virtue! Besides gender, of course, cultures too can differ (often greatly) in the degree of self-telling their members are allowed or encouraged. Certainly individuals differ as well, some more driven than others by the autobiographical imperative.

But, however much we may be conditioned *not* to know ourselves, we are also driven *to* know ourselves. From deep within even the prenarrative level of our lives surges some measure of the "urge to confess" (Pennebaker, 1990), the urge to lay out our lifestory in unedited, unexpurgated form (though language itself will *con*form our tale in socially sensible ways). Novelist John Cowper Powys describes this as "the universal craving to be listened to," which, "while we complain and explain, confess and excuse, narrate and recall soon sweeps away . . . all worrying speculation as to the impression produced by our monologue on the other person. Only to be heard!" Powys exclaims. "Only to fill the *whole* stage for one blessed interval!" (Blythe, 1979, p. 89).

As Powys implies, if this craving grows sufficiently intense, we may fear that once we get started we will be unable to stop: that once the sluiceway is opened, and all the hopes and hurts, opinions and obsessions, secrets and questions, worries and weird ideas—all the stuff of our inside story—come pouring out, we will overwhelm both ourselves and others in its wake. Nonetheless, we often (if not consciously) lace our speech with words like cancer or separated, or phrases like "that's another story," to entice our listener to get us to tell more of our tale. Thus, names dropped offhandedly, situations mentioned in passing, or scattered data about our ailments or achievements function like bits of hypertext on which our listener is (tacitly) invited to "click" and so penetrate more widely the web of our world.

Going from inside to inside-out in a way that satisfies this need to be known requires a different sort of listener from ones we might get in everyday life or were treated to as a child. Not someone who is forever correcting us or putting us down, or continually interrupting with *their* story instead, but a fair witness, someone who invites us to tell ourselves as deeply as we desire. In many respects, such a listener lies inside us already, a possibility we consider now in looking at two main ways of telling our lives—to ourselves and to others.

Telling Ourselves

We are constantly telling ourselves to ourselves. When awake, we narrate our lives *ad nauseam* in "an episodic, sometimes semi-conscious but virtually uninterrupted monologue" (Brooks, 1985, p. 13). When asleep, the telling continues in our dreams, albeit in jumbled or fantastic form. Unless we are focused on a particular task, however, much of this self-chatter, like the average conversation, is meandering in nature. Indeed, we are forever interrupting ourselves—our mind darting off in one direction after another, backward and forward in time, prompted by God knows what stimuli, natural or social.

Telling ourselves *intentionally* means directing this activity one word, one sentence at a time, according to the linear limitations of language itself (part of the "slippage" we noted in Chapter 3 that refracts our experience in the course of giving expression to the same). One method for doing so is keeping a journal. In a journal, one side of us (the narrator) tells ourselves to another side (the reader). In other words, there is always a someone to whom we do our telling, which points again to the rhetorical complexity of all self-telling. Thus, not just in writing a letter to someone else (which for some is a substitute for keeping a journal) but in keeping a diary for ourselves, we are never unaware of *audience*, of the "other" to whom our writing is done and of the voice it requires—or beguiles—us to adopt.

Though not every one of us will find journal keeping our forte (depending on our confidence in writing or our fear of exposure if our writings are read by the wrong eyes), it has benefits on a number of levels—psychologically, emotionally, relationally, even spiritually (see Rainer, 1978). In expressing our experience, it can accomplish a variety of purposes at the same time: purge troubling feelings, test out versions of particular events, identify issues for deeper probing, dream the future or dwell on the past; or nurse some silenced side of us till we can try it out in public. As such, a journal can be a vehicle for telling, reading, and *re*telling all at once.

Another method of telling ourselves to ourselves is compiling an autobiography. Much has been written on the various approaches we can take and emphases we can make: chronological order, particular themes, key relationships, major turning points, and so forth. Much has also been written on the rhetorical complexities, gendered constructions, and epistemological paradoxes of autobiography as a literary genre, in which, through language, the self simultaneously records, critiques, and creates—narrates, reads, and authors—itself (see Olney, 1980; LeJeune, 1989; Eakin, 1985; Smith, 1987; Heilbrun, 1988). It is not for us to exhaust these matters here, however, since they can sidetrack us from the path we are trying to steer in this book. Suffice it to say, writing an autobiography will also not be everyone's preference, for it requires not only time but self-esteem.

To some degree, we have to feel that our story is interesting, that we have something special to share with the world—some insight or wisdom that someone will deem worth reading. Feeling these things, however, places pressure on our task. Thus, many of us who might pour out our hearts in a journal balk at autobiography because we assume it a genre fit only for the famous. *Who would want to read the story of* my *little life?* we ask. As strategies for the telling phase of restorying our lives, as modes of autobiographical reflection, there are important differences, then, between keeping a journal and writing an autobiography. They concern both structure and audience.

Unless kept in accordance with a particular life-writing program (see Progoff, 1975), a journal is comparatively unstructured. Though conceivable as an autobiography-in-progress or as sketches for a more formal opus, it is essentially an ongoing repository of whatever strikes us as noteworthy amid the ever-changing fabric of our lives. Restricted only by the conventions of grammar and spelling, we can pick up on one event or emotion, one issue or idea, focus on it, and then move to another. In the course of fleshing out the significance of each, we will probably proceed in a meandering manner, reflective of the usual movements of consciousness itself—roaming now back into our past, now forward into our future, and now around us in the context of our present.

However, the restrictions of language are not to be ignored. In a journal, we may edit less fiercely than in an autobiography (as we shall see), but we edit nonetheless. We may strive for "stream of consciousness," but the mere act of putting thoughts into readable language always diverts the flow.

Moreover, while a journal is a record of our incessant inner "chattering" (Field, 1952), it can record only a portion at best. And to the portion we select to explore—the event that stands out, the question that persists, the theme that recurs—we may give inordinate attention, making more of it than perhaps *ought* to be made simply because the words seem easy to find. As we realize how much can thus be made from so tiny a segment of what swirls around inside, we may be overwhelmed by how much remains—how little of our lives we have noticed across the years, how little of our text we have taken the time to read. Hence the principle that the deeper we peer into the well of our soul, the more water we find, and the more unfathomable— and intriguing—we discover ourselves to be.

(Though perhaps more disturbing as well, since at the same time as we may get things off our chest, we may also stir things up, overwhelming ourselves with material that still causes pain—with story-lines that continue to trigger troubling emotions. For this reason, we may experience resistance to our self-telling that makes us decide not to go into certain things until we feel ready. For this reason also, gerontologists have found that the supposed *positive* effects of life review among the elderly are by no means universal (see Haight and Webster, 1995). In Chapter 6, we consider the ethical issues associated with this situation in terms of storylistening.)

An autobiography, on the other hand, imposes structure on a lived life. Whereas entries in a journal take the form that the spirit prescribes at the time, the material of our life as laid out in an autobiography must, like any extended literary work, assume a direction, selection, and coherence—that is, be plotted. For one thing, while there are many forms an autobiography can take, it must ultimately have a beginning, middle, and end—if only the arbitrary end of the moment we stop writing. But this simple requirement forces premature closure on our still unfolding experience, in the view of some critics making it epistemologically a suspect genre (see Olney, 1980). Related to the closure issue is the implicit pressure to construct a happy ending for ourselves, which means to portray the present as one in which we have "arrived" in some way, have acquired some solutions to the long standing issues of our life, or at least have summoned sufficient confidence to commit ourselves to write. As it were, there is pressure to get outside our own death, aesthetically speaking, and wrap our mind around the shape of our life before we have completely lived it.

These intrinsic, structural limitations on autobiography are not meant to discredit it as a means of self-creation. Indeed, for some it is nothing less than "an effort to find salvation, to make one's experience come out right, . . . to make a home for oneself, on paper" (Kazin, 1981, pp. 35, 42).

However, in a way more obvious than in keeping a journal, an autobiography must be laid out in a followable manner. Moreover, we cannot include whatever we wish. Our sense of audience, of the "other" who will someday read the record of our life—this, too, will censor our self-telling and edit its form.

Telling Others

Telling ourselves to others—not on paper but in person—is the second way of engaging in the first stage of restorying. It is integral to the kind of quality co-authoring we have been considering all along. Like journal keeping, it has a free-flowing aspect where we can tell whatever, and however, we wish. Two important differences, though, are that it is oral rather than literal and that it involves a fellow human being.

As for the oral dimension, *talking* ourselves inside-out is different from *writing* ourselves inside-out. We wield language, we swim in it, differently. We still textualize our lives explicitly, but we use a different medium to do so. Accordingly, we express a different message. Not only is the story*teller* not quite the same as the story*writer* but neither is the self that is spoken the same as the self that is written. (As we have seen, guided autobiography uses both media, yet the tension between orality and literacy goes back as far as Plato, so we shall not resolve it here [Havelock, 1991].) Moreover, people who tell themselves primarily through writing may relate to others in distinctive ways—may be more withdrawn from them, possibly, even more disdainful of them, as if the more they have confided to themselves on paper, the less they need to confide to others in person.

As for the audience dimension, when we keep a journal or write an autobiography we do so in private, without interference. Then, if we like, we can pass it onto someone else for feedback after the fact—which may stimulate a dialogue that starts another round of self-exploration on another, deeper level. But in telling ourselves to other people, our sense of who they are—how well they know us, how intelligent they are, how much they care—inevitably shapes our telling. We tell ourselves one way to a close friend, another to a therapist, and another to a stranger on the train. In psychoanalysis, this is known as *transference* (Spence, 1982). Just as we do not story ourselves in a vacuum, we cannot *tell* ourselves in a vacuum either. Our self-telling to each listener—no matter the nature of our relationship— will always be clean in some ways but cluttered in others. Like stories themselves, neither storytelling nor storylistening is ever innocent.

Also, to whomever we tell ourselves we tend to retain no permanent record of the text of our telling. We have only their memory of it and ours,

neither of which may be terribly accurate. Moreover, it is quickly susceptible to the distortions of storyotyping, both theirs of us and ours of ourselves—unless we make a tape of our telling, from which a transcript can
then be typed to augment (or stand against) our respective memories of the
oral one.

In future sections, we will say more about the complexity of listening
and the roles played in our restorying by the listeners to whom we tell
ourselves. For the moment, what is it that, in the telling phase, we should
be attempting to tell? The short answer is: anything and everything: whatever we *want* to tell or *can* tell. There ought to be no limits. If the narrative
environment provided by our listener is as blank, yet inviting, as a fresh
page in our journal, then no restrictions (except time) should apply. However, insofar as our goal is to articulate the text of our lifestory so that we
can read it and revise it *as a story*, we can focus on the same elements of
story we have considered before.

As for *plot*, we can try to identify the events that have figured thus far in
our life-course—what seem to be the main ones first, and the minor ones
next, plus the principal turning points. Moreover, we can focus on venting
some of the signature stories we listed for ourselves last chapter, then on as
many as we can of the other types and tidbits of our story material: short
and long, subplot and chapter, past *and future*. That is, we can dig into not
just our memories of what has been but our anticipations (hopes and fears)
of what may be, bearing in mind that, as a life*story,* we live "in the middest"
between our beginning and our end (Kermode, 1966).

As for *character*, we can try to get out of ourselves the history (at least
as we have constructed it) of the various people in our lives—major and
minor—and of our relationships with them, indulging ourselves as much as
we can in detailed description of their looks, their mannerisms, their way
with us, their lifestyles, and as much as we can imagine of their inner
thoughts and feelings.

As for *themes*, we can vary the strategy of guided autobiography to talk
out our ongoing experiences with such general matters as money, love,
death, sex, food, spirituality, and so on. This is an excellent approach for
grazing over the content of our inner story-world. However, as we shall
consider under Reading, there is merit in letting ourselves elaborate themes
that may be specific to us, that emerge from the text of our own life rather
than are prescribed for it by others (see Csikszentimihalyi and Beattie,
1979).

As for *setting*, we can tell about the geography of our lives, the physical
surroundings in which we have lived, the architecture of the buildings in

which we have worked or been sheltered across the years—how they each looked and felt. We can also get out of ourselves the different larger stories by which we have been shaped. We can start with our family story: going as far back into it as we can, even to past generations, taking care to identify its main events, central characters, key turning points, and so forth. Then, we can move to the community (or communities) in which we have been rooted, the creed that has structured our picture of the world, and each of the clubs, companies, or cultures that have stamped our lifestyle to any degree—recounting as much as we can about its history, about *our* history within it, and about our feelings concerning it.

The point in this first stage is not to analyze our lifestory, simply to *express* it as fully as we can. But even this is transformative. Getting ourselves out of ourselves, turning our inside text inside-out (on paper or in the ears of another), inevitably changes us. "We are simply more than we were before" (Winquist, 1980, p. 60). Going thus intentionally from experience to expression, we expand, we evolve. Like the chambered nautilus, we step outside of the same old story. No longer thus so stuck in particular interpretations of who we are, we open to the possibility that one life (our own) can have more than one version. We become—to ourselves—a different person, for the entire exercise both empties and fills.

On the one hand, it begins to purge us, even *exorcise* us, of the more troubling, less looked-at corners of our lives, of the stories we have habitually left untold. This could include our more meandering, less tellable tales, the kind we typically preface with "I'm afraid it's a rather *long* story"—the kind we have failed to get out in the past because we could never find the right words or the right frame of mind, or were afraid of them engulfing us with unresolved feelings, or were routinely interrupted from recounting by impatient listeners. On the other hand, getting these stories out can enhance our sense of substance. It can spawn respect for the vastness of our inner world, for the mass of unsavored stuff we have been storing (and re-storing) inside us but that now lies bubbling behind our eyes—more accessible than ever for conscious reflection. Finally, it can increase our personal power, not the *potential* power of the story left untold, but the *actual* power that every story, once aired, injects into the world.

Reading

"Most readers," observes one scholar, "*under*read"; "indeed, it is not uncommon for large parts of a novel to go virtually unread" (Kermode, 1980, p. 84). If we seldom ever tell ourselves in the fullblown ways just sketched, if we routinely under*tell* the text of our lives, it is easy to see why we might under*read* it as well. Tragically, this means we chronically underappreciate the interestingness, and depth, of our accumulated experience. It also means we fail to see either the opportunity or the means to restory. Thus, we stay mired in our story, hostages to its plot. But if reading literature has the potential to transform us, might not reading our *life*stories have similar power? This, then, is the double insight that ought to haunt us: first, the untold life is not open to being read; second, the unread life is not open to being restoried.

As we have seen, self-consciousness is rhetorically complex. To our own lifestory, we are several selves at once: author, narrator, protagonist, and reader. In relation to any text, however, the functions of author and reader are closely entwined. The reader of a text is in some way its author as well, insofar as in the act of reading he or she creates the meaning the text may mediate. Reading is thus authoring—just as, from another angle, authoring is reading. This has led one scholar, Roland Barthes, to proclaim "the death of the author" ([1968] 1990). Though there are nuances in this reader-author equation that are beyond our mandate here, we can venture at least this: in reading ourselves to the degree we encourage in what follows, we are effectively taking greater authorship of our lives, opening ourselves to fresh and freeing interpretations of who we are and what we can be.

The stage of reading, then, is the stage of stepping back from the text of our lives as we have begun to lay it out and critiquing it with dispassionate yet affectionate concern—as we might a beloved piece of literature: *This is my lifestory, yes. But what do I make of it?* Where in the first stage we explicitly textualize our life, in this one we explicitly analyze that text. Where the first stage was a deliberate *de*-storying, a shedding of our narrative skin, this is a deconstructing (or *de*-composing) of what we have made of ourselves to date. It is a particular type of "editing," more formal and focused than the summarizing we do each day.

Reading our life-text need not be separate, timewise, from telling it. In fact, telling, reading, and *re*telling overlap continually. Nonetheless, reading ourselves *as composed* is a distinct task, for we are changing our point of view. Just as in the telling phase we move from self-as-character (caught *in* our lifestory) to self-as-narrator, so in this phase we move from self-as-narrator to self-as-reader. This is a significant shift. We can think of our experience with a piece of fiction. The story the narrator tells us is not the same as what we *re*tell, in our own words. We can never quite capture the range of emotions and associations conjured up as we read, few of which, in turn, will be exactly what the author intended to evoke. Depending how deeply we engaged in the reading, we will feel different feelings, draw different conclusions, and infer different meanings.

Every day, of course, we all make such shifts in perspective. At some juncture we all step back from ourselves. Just as we tell ourselves on a regular basis, so do we read ourselves—to figure out our lives: what this means, what that means. None of us lives the unexamined life completely. None of us is entirely unreflective, uncritical of our actions or words, decisions or feelings—nor those of others. Indeed, we commonly refer to trying to "read" other people to figure *them* out: their body language, their motives and moods. Some of us, brought up in family stories under an authoritarian parent, can become so skilled—for survival's sake—at reading the texts of others' lives (what they are going to do next, etc.) that we are lost when invited to read our own. Or we can become paranoid, reading into ordinary events far more than seems justified or sane. Thus, some of us read our lives too little and others too much. However, we are all readers to some degree.

But in intentionally self-reading, what are we reading *for*? The answer is not simple, since reading per se is a complex process. As to what it is, how reading written texts differs from reading oral ones, and how the act of reading itself, as well as the content being read, changes the reader—little is definitively known, despite the fact that humans have been reading texts, fictional or not, written or not, since the invention of language.

From their study of readers' responses to literary texts, researchers Hunt and Vipond (see Beach, 1990) have found, however, that readers (at least of fiction) fall into three main types: First, those who are "point-driven," who look at the central concept, or moral, of the story; second, those who are "information-driven"; third, those who are "story-driven," whose primary agenda is "reading for the plot" (Brooks, 1985). It seems fair to add that there are readers who are *atmosphere*-driven as well (for whom a story is more alluring for its overall "feel" than for how it turns out); or *character*-driven (for whom how characters are developed is more important than the sequence of events); or *meaning*-driven. In this last, readers read for aspects of the story that are behind it, as it were, or between the lines. They read for the point of the story not so much for its own sake as for them and their world.

What we have been implying in this book is that different people, with varying storying styles, tend to read their *life*stories for particular reasons. However, to appreciate their full range of aesthetic possibilities, it is crucial to try reading for all of these reasons. "Rereading the plot of your life," as one journaling expert advises (Rainer, 1978), is valuable for discerning the trajectory of our life's events, past through present to future, and for assessing the selection and coherence we have imposed on our experience in the course of textualizing it. But so is reading for the characterizations by which we have lived—of others and of ourselves. So, too, is reading for atmosphere, for themes (as we saw with guided autobiography), and for meaning.

As we hinted in Chapter 2, the meaning of *meaning* in story terms is difficult to explain, which means that the question of meaning in *life*story terms may resist a precise answer. Nonetheless, it is a pivotal concept for any form of therapoeisis. In the storytelling-storylistening exchange of psychoanalysis, for example, reading for meaning is central. Says Spence (1982), the "search after meaning" is "the analyst's stock in trade" (p. 107), with the goal being "to turn the patient's life into a meaningful story" (p. 123). The problem, though, is that there is no *one* meaning to be found. As McAdams puts it, "if lives are like texts, then lives, too, have no inherent meanings" (1994, p. 781). Like a good novel, there is no end to the meanings we can pull from a life. Thus, though our lifestories have no *particular* meanings, they are infinitely meaning-*ful*. They are truly open books—like the best literature, and people, to which we can be exposed. Furthermore, because we are still moving into our own future (since our lifestory is not complete), the present perspective from which we analyze our past experience is itself forever shifting, forever advancing. "Because life is unfinished," says Kerby, "so is the meaning of the past" (1991, p. 31).

What we read our lives *for*, then, are the same sorts of things we have been discussing all along: the elements of story. Accordingly, a number of questions can be asked of our life-text by way of critiquing it *as a story*—questions we can ask, by ourselves, of the written text of our journal or autobiography, or, with a listener, of the oral one. Since we have already identified many of these questions in previous chapters, we shall repeat only the more obvious ones here.

As you will see, however, we have worded these questions in a somewhat detached manner, much as might a literary critic in focusing less on the life of the author than on the text his or her imagination has produced. Furthermore, it is unnecessary to ask these questions in order. Any of them can be played with at any time, depending on our interest and what we and our listener find worth pursuing. Any one represents a way into the heart of our whole life-text. All lead sooner or later to the same deeper understanding into how we have composed our life thus far and might want to re-compose it in the future.

They lead, that is, not into the past (or future) per se but into the stories we have made of it; not the past (or future) as it is, but as we have textualized it. To ask them is thus to focus not on the content of our life-story material as much as on the *form* in which it is conveyed—the form of our self-telling. This means playing literary *theorist* of our life-text more than literary critic (Chatman, 1978). It also means examining the relationship between the form of our life *as told* to its form *as lived*. Finally, it means our focus is like that of the young Robert Coles (1989, p. 23), whose mentor during his residency in psychiatry "urged [him] to be a good listener [of his patients] in the special way a story requires: note the manner of presentation; development of plot, character; the addition of new dramatic sequences; the emphasis accorded to one figure or another in the recital; and the degree of enthusiasm, of coherence, the narrator gives to his or her account."

Since it is a huge task to tackle the entire text we have told during the telling stage, one solution, to start, is to focus on the texts of some of our signature stories instead (see "Bill's Iron Lung Story" in Chapter 3). Signature stories, you will recall, can be viewed as parables that reveal much about how we see ourselves in the midst of our lives, of others' lives, and of our ultimate environment. Though they provide a limited amount of lifestory material, they can be said to represent that material in miniature. Analyzing them both individually and collectively can thus turn up broad trends in the *form* (as much as the *content*) of our self-telling that can be reflected on and then looked for in our other material as well. In this way, we move from the microscopic perspective on our lives to the macro one.

After giving such a close reading to a number of our signature stories, and to as much as we can of the rest of the material we have told, we might then step back from our whole narrative corpus and pose of it the following general questions:

- Are there any broad patterns in these various pieces of lifestory material—in terms of plot, character, point of view, theme, genre, and setting? What are they? How is this material connected? Taken together, does it tell a single, overriding story? What is it? What is its plot line overall? the *shape* of our life as a whole? And what type of story is it?

- What sorts of things have got included in this material? What, excluded? What does this say to us? How do we feel about the material we have included? about what we have edited out? about the stories we have left untold? What does this say about how we have storied our life thus far? about our storying style? How do we feel about this?

- Of which of our stories are we specially fond? Why? Which could we not do without? Why? Which could we drop from our collection? Why? If we could change our collection of stories in any way, what would it be? Why? Are there other stories we would *like* to be able to tell about ourselves? What are they?

- What would we say is the relationship between the stories we tell inside-out and the full sweep of our outer existence? of our inner experience? of the stories others appear to have of us outside-in? What gaps are there between these various levels? What do we make of them? What do they mean?

After asking such questions of our library of lifestory material, we can move to reading the larger stories that have shaped us overall—for example, our family of origin, the family we have created or married into, our marriage itself, our close friendships, each of the clubs, communities, institutions, and organizations in which we have been involved. After listing what these stories are, we might *rank* them in order of their impact upon our life—emotionally, intellectually, philosophically, sociologically, spiritually, interpersonally, and so forth. As we approach this part of the reading process, it might help to remind ourselves that, metaphorically, these stories comprise the *setting* of our lifestory. Thinking of each as having its particular poetic structure, narrative environment, and approach to coauthoring, we can start, then, with the one we rank highest and ask such questions as:

- What sort of role(s) have we played in this larger story? What sort of character have we been—flat/round, major/minor? How have others tended to characterize us? How fully and fairly have they seen the real us? What sort of storyotyping have they indulged in toward us? How has this felt?

- What have been the main events in this larger story? What have been its turning points, main conflicts, central characters, stated and underlying themes, guiding myths? Finally, how has our personal lifestory been influenced by each of these aspects?

- What code of telling and listening did we learn in the narrative environment of this larger story? How was it communicated or taught? What forms of self-telling tended to be encouraged? discouraged? How did this feel?

- What is/was the authority structure in this larger story? How is/was it enforced? What is/was our response to it? How much authority have we had over our own lifestory within this larger story? How do we feel about this? What changes would we like to make in this regard? Why? What kind and quality of coauthoring have we experienced in this larger story? with what effect on us?

- What view of ourselves and our world—what philosophy of life—has this larger story instilled in us? In what ways? How effectively? How deeply has its story-world affected us? How do we feel about this?

Asking such questions of both our lifestories and the larger stories in which they are set allows us a critical detachment from our lives as we have constructed them thus far. Ideally, it increases both our objectivity about them and our affection for them. It should also increase our sense of how they might have been—and can still be—different from what they are. It ought to heighten our sense of possibility—as opposed to facticity—in composing our lives, a process we can now claim with a more authoritative sense of our own agency (White and Epston, 1990). So it is that we turn to the third stage of restorying: *retelling* our lives.

Retelling

Telling and living are tightly entwined. Writes Carr, "we are constantly striving . . . to occupy the story-teller's position with respect to our own actions" (1986, p. 60). The ways we narrate ourselves to both ourselves and others (though there are generally gaps between the two) are inseparable from our emotions, our relationships, our whole mode of being in the world. Says William Bridges, "each person's life is a story that is telling itself in the living" (1980, p. 71). Having told and read our life as intensively as we have now done, having effectively transcended our story as hitherto composed, we are ready to make decisions concerning how to compose it from now on. There are a number of things to bear in mind, however, as we enter this final stage of the restorying process.

The first concerns *resistance*. Retelling our lives is easier said than done, for to retell them is effectively to re-*form* them, on several levels at once—not just cognitively but emotionally, behaviorally, interpersonally, ethically, and ontologically. This can mean radical change, something we may not rush to embrace. Such resistance can come not just from others, though (for as *we* restory they may have to as well), but also from ourselves. Its strength will be proportionate to the tie between how we tell our lives and how we live them. And they have to be tied a little; otherwise, we are in a state of self-deception—a divided state indeed, though in reach of us all.

The second thing is that retelling takes time, more time than telling and reading together. This is because it requires stepping back still further from the text of our lives than we have done in telling and reading it, with the goal of not only *having* a new story but *being* one as well. Retelling thus entails asking ourselves what changes we would like to make, what new interpretations to try in old situations. Furthermore, as we see how event by event, and overall, a different story can better account for the same events, then all things begin to be made new. Such a *de*-storying of ourselves requires not just time, therefore, but also courage, for we are stepping into a brave new story-world. Constructing such a world—in memory, relationship, *and action*—cannot happen overnight. Moreover, insofar as our old ways of self-telling are "recipes for structuring experience itself, for laying down routes into memory" (Bruner, 1987, p. 31), we cannot expect to uproot these routes and replace them all at once. Our characteristic storying style has had a lifetime to become entrenched in—and *as*—our soul.

Third, retelling requires attention to language, to the actual words with which we tell ourselves who we are and what is going on. It may mean learning a new vocabulary, a new set of phrases and terms—for example, shifting from "you" (or blaming) statements to "I feel" ones that signify our ownership of the ways we *construct* situations, other people's actions and reactions, and so forth; and embracing more affirmative phrases for describing ourselves, like differently-abled rather than crippled, or creative as opposed to stupid or dumb. It also means paying attention to the *sub*-text of our self-telling, to what we communicate between the lines of what we say and do. It requires vigilance regarding the genre in which we habitually describe situations, turn events into experiences, and lay down our memories, an awareness of the point of view with which we usually narrate ourselves. In all, it involves recognizing our unique voice amid the cacophony of others', becoming familiar with its sound, and testing it in the world.

Fourth, retelling requires sensitivity to the interpretations placed on the events of our lives not only by ourselves but by others as well. It means being aware of the various narrative environments within which we live (or have lived) and the forms of self-telling they encourage and discourage, plus being deliberate about not falling into them again. It thus means resisting the authority of others *over* us, questioning their storyotypes *of* us, and challenging the interpretations they routinely place *for* us on our actions and intentions, on what we have done in the past and should do in the future.

Fifth, then, retelling can entail actually *changing* narrative environments, or re-contextualizing our lives. This could involve something obvious like leaving home, or, if we have the means, moving to a different community and, storywise, starting afresh. As social creatures, in other words, we may need new *coauthors* to help us make new meanings. This is where a support group enters in—new people (and potentially friends) to evoke different versions of familiar situations, to help us move beyond thinking and feeling according to "the same old story," and to adjust the dominant genre through which we make sense of events—say, from tragedy to adventure, or from seeing difficult situations as reasons for mourning to celebrating them as occasions for learning.

Sixth, retelling means looking at the material we have typically left untold, revisiting parts of our experience that our expression has overlooked, and speculating on parts of our existence that we failed to experience the first time around. As White and Epston (1990) say, "persons are rich in lived experience" (our term for existence) but "only a fraction of this experience can be storied and expressed at any one time." However, "those aspects of [it] that fall outside of the dominant story provide a rich and fertile source for the generation, or re-generation, of alternative stories" (p. 15).

Different though it be from the old one, though, the new overriding version we begin to weave of ourselves—past, present, and future—must still be accountable to the facts of our existence, or to our facticity. Not any old story will do. While we are surely free to compose ourselves, we cannot make ourselves up however we wish (Polonoff, 1987)—cannot become imposters to our own selves, as it were. The other people in our lives, provided we do not change social circles completely, will be sure to keep us in check in this regard. At the first hint of our acting out of character, they are likely to snap us back to reality, or at least to the role in terms of which they have characterized us thus far, which is "reality" for them.

In this book, however, we deliberately offer no answer to the overall question as to which direction we ought to restory. Instead, our belief is that the more we tell and read the text of our lives, the more that direction will reveal itself on its own; our unique inner wisdom will be freer to be our guide. Mystical as this sounds, there can be no cookie-cutter patterns, no prepackaged analytical schemas, with which to story our lives. Ultimately, we are novel. We alone can judge. Only thus can the story we live be *our* story, our *whole* story, and *nothing but* our story.

Restorying is thus something we ourselves can direct. We may draw on outer resources as they apply, but we need not surrender our authorship to others, whether an individual like a therapist, parent, or spouse; a collective such as our clan or creed; or a program that would push its preferred formula, template-like, for making sense of our lives. No one but ourselves can tell us who we are, or who we can become. The onus is on us. Within the rich, sprawling text of our own infinitely interpretable experience we hold whatever answers we need and wisdom we seek. These precious things lie within us, not without; they cannot be prescribed by others, only discovered by ourselves (see Randall and Kenyon, in preparation). Should we fail to explore this meaning and express this wisdom, however, that text is a wasted resource, unhonored by ourselves and unavailable to others whose lives it might enrich, like a great story that hides unwritten in the soul of a novelist who lacks the courage to get it out.

RESTORYING EACH OTHER'S LIVES

Storywise, none of us is an island. Not only are our individual lifestories emplotted in a complex web of larger stories, but they are enmeshed with the lifestories of numerous others. As Tennyson says, "I am a part of everything I have met." For this reason, stimulating and steering the restorying process is not the sole province of professional life-change experts. On the contrary: for better or worse, we are continually coauthoring each other in the course of composing our lives. Accordingly, we wish now to highlight the roles we can play for one another as agents of restorying—whether formally, in a counseling relationship, or informally, by means of intimacy or friendship, both short term and long.

A basic conviction among adult educators is that a teacher should be not a "sage on the stage" but a "guide on the side." As coauthors of each other's lives, it is this latter role we play, what we referred to before as biographical coach. Guide is acceptable because it is possible, as a friend of ours once commented, to get *lost* in our own story. We frequently need a companion to journey with us through the cloud of unknowing that can enshroud our lives, for we are complex creatures, inside and out. There is no way to know ourselves completely, to get to the end of our lifestory and experience the conclusion and confirmation—the resolution and revelation—that endings intrinsically confer. We are constantly changing. The emplotment of our lives can never keep pace with their development (Hillman, 1975). Furthermore, our lifestories are never true, as in accurate or clear, but multilayered and susceptible to several versions. Though the onus is on us, the task of interpreting who we are is too vast and befuddling to be tackled *entirely* unaided.

Guide *on the side* is the key, however, because we have no right to assume we can be up ahead leading the way for our partner along the path of *his or her* self-creation, as if scouting out territory he or she is incapable of exploring alone. Quite the contrary. Only he or she is positioned to proceed through the maze of his or her own memory and imagination; to enter his or her "true novel" and discover the wealth of story material, the sacred text, that comprises his or her soul.

We also have no right to assume, as some in the helping professions can seem to, that we can be present to other persons storyless ourselves. We have our own lifestory; however much we submerge it or ignore it, it is there.

It does not magically disappear. Through it, we hear them telling theirs. In the process, we inevitably characterize them, even storyotype them, on the strength of what we hear—and see. As we argue in the next chapter, however, we can nonetheless try to be open to what, amid *our* lifestory, we can learn from them amid theirs, and what we can learn from *their* restorying as we, presumably, continue ours. In this way, the restorying is more mutual, and none of us has special authority with respect to the others. Not that we must never say what we think when asked for our advice, or have no authority to contribute at all, but that our use of this authority is expressed by *with* rather than *over*, and thus by the prefix *co-*.

In the telling phase of the restorying process, we are listeners—or *co*-auditors—to the tale they are getting out, the principle being that when we *tell* ourselves, part of us *hears* ourselves, too. In the reading phase, we are critics—or *co*-editors—of the lifestory they are critiquing with a scrutiny perhaps never before applied. In the third phase, we are authors—or *co*-authors—as they test out new ways of telling who they are: interpreting their life-events along different plot lines and according to different genres, and using different characterizations of both others and themselves. And as they attempt to implement these new ways of composing their lives, we "stick around" (Kegan, 1982, p. 121) as a more supportive "narrative environment" than they have enjoyed with others in their past—the harbinger, hopefully, of what they can enjoy in the future.

Of course, there is no reason why we would ever be the sole co-auditor, -editor, and -author for any one person as he moves through the stages of restorying, nor he for us. Indeed, we frequently catch each other at different points in this never-ending process—cycle, really, since once begun it tends to repeat itself, spiraling ever further from telling through reading to retelling, and on to telling again. Thus, we sometimes happen upon individuals in the telling phase—when we are the stranger-on-the-train for them, for instance—yet after we leave the train, there is no way to continue with them through the reading and retelling. That role may fall to someone else. Other times, we may (quite unwittingly) play co-editor as someone tests out different versions of her lifestory and examines how she has composed it up to now, having vented it initially to another listener's ear.

This underlines the mystery of being human. We never fully know how we affect each other's lives. We can never anticipate what "butterfly effect" may be set off down a whole chain of people by a single smile or frown. We often help each other restory in powerful ways without ever realizing it. But perhaps it is not important to realize it, to feel consciously that we are instrumental—or, God forbid, indispensable—in another person's restorying. If we did, we might make ourselves paranoid about the ripple effects, storywise, of our every word and deed in the lives of those we touch. Perhaps it is more important simply to be *open* to being whatever we can in our encounters with others, regardless of where they are on the road of restorying, and open to receiving the same on the path of our own.

STRATEGIES FOR STORYLISTENING

We are talking here about "the other side of the story" of the restorying process—the side of storylistening. As the saying goes, "you can't tell who you are unless someone is listening" (Keen and Fox, 1974, p. 9). Before we consider the ethical aspects of such listening in the next chapter, however, we want to offer some practical strategies that, in the spirit of those offered to Coles (1989), will help us appreciate the literary and textual dimensions of another's lifestory, while respecting its inseparability from his or her life. Whenever other people enter our presence, that is, all they bring to us *are* their stories. All we have to work with are ultimately texts—as experienced inside themselves, as expressed to us inside-out (in both actions and words), and as reconstructed (and summarized) by our own imagination outside-in, as our impression of who they are. Learning to listen *to* these multilayered texts—and listening to learn *from* them—is essential to coauthoring.

As Spence has shown concerning not only transference but also *counter*-transference in psychoanalysis, however, all listening is refracted by the hidden agenda, the *sub*text, of the listener's own lifestory. Again, we listen *through* our lifestories, never around them. Nonetheless, it is always possible to improve our listening skills. By adapting the following strategies to our unique listening style, we can become more compassionate agents of growth in others' lives. In the warm phrase of Robert Atkinson (1995), we shall be "giving [them] their lifestory," an essentially *sacred* act. Furthermore, we shall be helping to foster a narrative environment in the midst of everyday life that is more conducive to our collective self-creation because calmer and quieter. In other words, if all of us were listened to better perhaps we might talk a lot less; perhaps we rattle on as much as we can because we feel listened to so little.

1. Listen with respect for the novelty of the other person's lifestory, for the rich texture of his* unique tale. Listen with openness for how interesting he really is, and let him know you find him so (for this itself can empower a person).

*For the sake of both gender balance and reading ease, we have alternated the use of masculine and feminine pronouns from one strategy to the next.

Listen despite the storyotypes you are bound to build around him. In other words, listen for the ways that his story is sure to press buttons in yours, but resist reacting in your usual way because of that. This means: Be in touch with the vastness and complexity of your own story, and be open to learning more about it as you learn about his.

2.   Listen with respect for the power of respectful, nonjudging listening to open a space for her to restory in safety, to find new meanings in her own lifestory material, and to test out a different version of herself from what she has told—and lived—in the past. At the same time, listen with respect for the resistance she may have to being listened to, for her resistance to being restoried. And listen with respect for the direction that she, not you, wants to go with the telling. Be mindful of the fact that in letting you listen at all, she is trusting you enough to let you hear her tale.

3.   Listen for the form of his self-telling as much as for its content. Do not get so caught up with the content that you miss the form. Listen for *how* he talks about himself as much as for *what* he says. Listen for the actual words he uses, the tell-tale expressions, the vocabulary and tone, the recurring metaphors and figures of speech. Listen for the genre in which the telling seems to be done, for his characteristic storying style, and for the ways his words are reinforced (or belied) by his gestures, actions, or eyes.

4.   Listen for how she characterizes herself, as well as others, amidst the circumstances and relationships she relates. Listen for hints of the guiding myth that underlies her sense of self. Listen for the themes that run through her anecdotes, and how these are handled, the philosophy of life to which they point.

5.   Listen for the plot lines by which the events he recounts are connected, the main turning points on which they turn, and the conflicts they reflect. Listen for the *sub*-plot lines and even *counter*-plot lines that run through his accounts. Listen for how such elements—plot, theme, character, genre—interact and intertwine in both the telling and (possibly) the living of his life.

6.   Listen for clues concerning the different larger stories in which her personal one has been set. Listen for indications of the particular poetic structure, narrative environment, and kind of coauthoring that have been characteristic of each, for how these have shaped her values and views and directed or restricted her self-creation. Listen for the key events and characters, the conflicts and turning points, that have been pivotal in each.

7.   Listen for what he does *not* say as much as for what he does, though listen with respect and not to pry. Listen for what is in the silences: the missing details, the omitted events, the unmentioned characters and themes—and be alert to the significance of such omissions, for the "narrative secrets" to which they might point. Listen for the stories he leaves untold, for the holes in his stories, for the stories within his story, for the one story behind the many, for the text beneath the text, or the *sub*text. Listen for the hints of other stories that could

be told if properly, and respectfully, coaxed. Listen for the stories he *likes* to tell—his signature stories—and those he keeps to himself. Above all, listen for the emotions that are in his story, and the stories that are behind his emotions.

8. Listen not to change her lifestory or fix it, which could be to wrest it unfairly from her and, in a sense, *de*-story her. Rather, listen to enlarge her story, to expand and deepen it, in this way "releasing the energy bound within it" (Houston, 1987, p. 99) and helping to increase her respect for her own storied depths.

9. Listen with concern to elicit less the "true" story than a coherent or plausible one. Do not disregard the truth issue entirely, but be aware that (historical) truth is in any case not attainable, and that even if it were, it is ultimately not as relevant as narrative truth. In other words, his lifestory, even if it plays loose with what you guess to be the facts, can still be the vehicle of truth, though of the type we encounter in a movie or novel or dream—a point one Alzheimer researcher has convincingly stressed (Crisp, 1995). At the same time, listen with alertness for the inevitable gaps between the levels of his lifestory—outside, inside, and so on—or between what he tells you with his words and, again, shows you with his gestures, actions, or eyes.

10. Listen for the type and degree of meaning-making she is inclined, or can be encouraged, to do. Listen with a view to helping her find more and newer meanings than she has made in the past, aware that her life, like any good story, is infinitely meaning*ful*.

11. Listen less for the facts of his life than for the interpretations he place upon them. And listen for the beginnings of different, possibly more positive interpretations, for alternative versions (*sub*-versions), that may be trying to break out between the lines of what he is saying, versions that you could midwife into being, thus putting a perhaps previously unimagined spin on the stuff of his life, which means opening the door for a new version of who he is.

12. Finally, listen not just to help *her* learn, but to learn *from her* yourself. Listen with openness for the message, wisdom, or truth that her life—as text and as told—uniquely embodies. Listen in awe of the fact that in the exchange between you, a new lifestory, and thus a new life, is being coauthored—both for her and, potentially, for you.

CONCLUSION

Restorying never stops. All of us restory constantly, if only in the subtle ways by which our picture of ourselves (and our world) gradually changes and expands. Some of us restory more dramatically, though over a lengthy period, while a few restory rather dramatically rather fast. To restory our lives in these latter, more intentional ways is, in a sense, to become a different person, which can be unsettling both for us and for those with whom we live. It is unsettling, yet unavoidable, for there is a call within us, whose source is ultimately unknown, that lures us toward a lifestory that is progressively bigger and better, more embracing of our actual existence. We have called that call the autobiographical imperative, and the process of responding to it, composing our lives.

We can let that process happen willynilly or take authority for it ourselves—and engage in it together, which may even speed it up. That is, as we get better at coauthoring each other, we may find the pace of our restorying accelerating until it becomes a way of life. It is like a chain: a different lifestory issues in different emotions, which lead to different actions, relationships, and commitments. All are connected. It is also like a circle, a hermeneutic circle. The more fully we are able to tell, then the more meaningful the reading we can do and the more we are enabled to *re*tell and *re*live. That restorying thus never ends may seem a terrible fate—to have no final answer (Schafer, 1989). But it is surely far less terrible a fate for it never to end than never to begin.

In this chapter, our focus has been on how to assume more authority for composing our lives. Whether we want them to or not, our experiences within the realm of education authorize us. So do those within religion. Art can authorize us as well—as can other people. But within the web of all these influences we can also authorize ourselves, and *co*-author one another. In the chapter we move to now, our focus is on the ethical issues that are at stake as we thus usher each other to greater growth by both storytelling and storylistening.

Chapter 6

Storytelling and Storylistening: Ethical Issues[1]

I've found that we feel stronger and more hopeful after writing and sharing our autobiographies. We see that we must have been good travellers to have gotten this far.

James Birren (1987)

INTRODUCTION

So far we have discussed the basic and intimate relationship that exists between our lifestories, ourselves, and each other. We have also considered in detail the ways in which we are stories and the process of changing our stories, personally and interpersonally. However, the intimacy and potential effectiveness of the stories we are urges us to consider the ethical issues associated with autobiographical reflection and restorying.

There are a number of significant ethical issues relevant to the life-as-story metaphor. It is interesting to note at the outset that some of the dilemmas with which we are concerned are not unique to the stories we are. However, the focus on stories and such things as biographical aging makes these issues that much more intense and significant: conversely, the discussion of specific ethical concerns provides another perspective on the value of studying the storied aspects of human nature.

We will deal with three ethical issues. First, we will address the idea of informed consent, as it applies in selected storylistening situations involving both research and practice. Second, we will consider an example of when storytelling and storylistening is necessary; that is, when people have a right to have someone listen to their story. And third, we will consider three guidelines for effective and responsive storylistening, as well as the dilemma of involvement. As we proceed through these sections, we will also be exploring the overall ethical issue of when to story and when not to story. As we have indicated throughout this volume, the examples we provide reflect our specific expertise and background, and therefore in this chapter are drawn largely from gerontology. However, we feel that the principles discussed and the insights gained apply more generally. Before we discuss the ethical issues themselves, a few remarks about ethics are in order.

STORYTELLING AND PRACTICAL ETHICS

The moral domain that interests us is that of *practical* ethics, in contrast to *theoretical* ethics (Kenyon and Davidson, 1993; Singer, 1979). Theoretical ethics deals with such things as the meaning of ethical concepts, including *autonomy* or freedom, and *beneficence* or doing no harm. While there is an overlap between these two types of ethics, practical ethics is a form of reasoning, a reflective process that attempts to answer the basic question, "what should I do in this situation, all things considered?" Practical ethics is the domain of action—moreover, action concerned with our own life or other people's lives.

Decision making in practical ethics is inherently complex, since it must take into consideration the interests of all persons directly or indirectly involved in a situation or affected by a course of action. This is what is meant by the phrase "all things considered." Ethical reasoning involves the attempt to put ourselves in another person's place and to see the larger picture, one that transcends self-interests, narrowly defined. It is a feature of ethics that it cannot be forced; it is a question of intentions and is firmly rooted in our freedom to choose and to care. We can all think of examples where people make it look as if they are behaving ethically, by virtue of the outside story they tell, when they are actually engaged in exploitation or manipulation on the inside. We cannot always tell what is going on in many situations. Nevertheless, ethics invites us to consider our policies, programs, and personal and professional behavior in a light that encompasses political, economic, scientific, and other more specific forms of reasoning. You could say it urges us to again acknowledge the larger story we live within.

INFORMED AND NEGOTIATED CONSENT

A basic ethical requirement of any storytelling, storylistening exchange—or what can be termed a *biographical encounter*—whether it be in the context of research or intervention, is the establishment of informed consent. This may not be a simple matter with many forms of biographical or qualitative research. It has been pointed out, for example, that professional codes of practice are not likely to provide sufficient guidelines in these cases. Kayser-Jones and Koenig (1994, p. 18) note that "the consent process is sometimes a prolonged negotiation between researcher and informants rather than a formalized moment at one point in time when a consent document is signed by an informant."

Informed consent in these situations amounts to an ethical imperative to establish mutual trust between researcher and/or practitioner and narrator or storyteller. The trust permits the storylistener to gather sometimes intimate information from the storyteller, but it also creates a moral obligation to ensure that the information does not create negative experiences or harm the participant and that the privileged position of access granted the storylistener will not be used to the participant's detriment.

Informed consent also involves rights to privacy and confidentiality on the part of the narrator, and the storylistener's responsibility to ensure the same. As examples, this is essential when accounts are published as citations in research journals or in books for the general public, and when they are stored in medical or psychological data banks (Ruth and Kenyon, 1996). As Fischer (1994, p. 4) notes in the context of research, "Social research holds out the promise of anonymity for respondents, but detailed individual stories may violate this promise." This is a serious ethical issue since storytellers are often relating pieces of their lifestories, for example, about intimate relationships between spouses or in families, that may never have been disclosed to another person.

In storytelling situations, informed consent is perhaps more appropriately termed *negotiated consent* (Moody, 1988), in that it reflects an ongoing process from the beginning to the completion of the biographical encounter. For example, while obtaining written consent for future uses of biographical materials is increasingly required by granting agencies, not all potential uses may be known at the outset of the encounter. If a different use arises, the researcher—or, say, a practitioner who wishes to write a book about his or her professional experiences—has an ethical obligation to contact the persons involved, if they are still living, and otherwise their families, before extensive documents of their lives are published. This point applies importantly to semiofficial or public use of psychiatric or medical data that are used after the fact, so to speak, and perhaps only remotely connected to the original purpose of data collection. As the information highway approaches being an information freeway, we cannot overestimate the importance of ethical dialogue on these issues. A right to privacy means that we have control over when and how communication about ourselves, or pieces of our story, are given to others, and confidentiality implies that an agreement has been made that limits access to that private information.

CONSENT AND COMPETENCE

Another subject of ethical discourse concerns the notion of informed consent as it applies to persons with specialized competence or varying degrees of *decisional capacity*. The important ethical dilemma here centers on the avoidance of two extremes. On the one hand, it is unethical to automatically rule out such persons from biographical forms of research and intervention, even if there is a degree of, for example, cognitive impairment. On the other hand, a person's capacity to make informed decisions needs to be assessed, and that assessment needs to be based on more than standard instruments, since those instruments themselves may be morally questionable in terms of their impact on a person.

The point here is that the assessment of competence itself may cause a person anxiety and loss of dignity—for example, in situations where dementing persons cannot identify pictures of ordinary objects and become self-conscious and embarrassed by the assessment process. What is necessary here is something in addition to standard instruments and risk-benefit analyses which, by themselves, only look at the person from the outside. Perhaps we need to use storytelling and storylistening as an integral part of the entire process. This is a particularly delicate and complex issue which requires sensitivity to particular situations. We will discuss the issue of competence in more detail in the following sections (see also Kayser-Jones and Koenig, 1994).

Voluntary Consent

A final question of concern with respect to informed consent is that of ensuring that it is truly voluntary, as it should be from an ethical perspective. This issue arises in the contexts of both research and practice. To take one example, the use of living wills and advance directives is increasing at a rapid rate. Further, residents of nursing homes and other institutions are being offered opportunities to complete such documents. While many people agree that these documents are designed to ensure autonomy and dignity on the part of older (and younger) persons, there is a danger that they can be implemented inappropriately.

As with other situations of this type, older persons in particular are at risk of inadvertent coercion through such things as a perceived fear of reprisal on the part of their caregivers and perhaps family members, or low self-esteem as a result of ageism. A suggested ethically appropriate alternative is an autobiographical approach to the implementation of advance directives which "means being prepared to take time both in educating respondents about the implications of their decisions, and in allowing their reflection to give rise to authentic choices" (Boetzkes, 1993, p. 450). Another way to say this is that informed or negotiated consent must be based clearly on a process of *personal storytelling*. A further implication of this view is that the professionals or others who introduce such documents need to be effective storylisteners and may themselves require specific training in this area.

WHEN STORYLISTENING IS NECESSARY

An important implication of the view that storytelling is an existential-spiritual phenomenon, as we have discussed throughout this volume, is that all persons, frail or well, are stories, are still creating stories, and have a story to tell. Thus, a dementing or otherwise frail person who resides in a nursing home, for example, should be considered to be more than, borrowing from Gubrium (1993), *a face without a story*. Rather, a frail older person should be considered to be *biographically active* and therefore a legitimate candidate for biographical intervention in such contexts as assessment and diagnosis in a hospital (Davidson, 1991), assessments of competence (Checkland and Silberfeld, 1993; Harrison, 1993), and community care (Gearing and Coleman, 1996). Frail older persons should also be eligible for various forms of therapy, including life-review and reminiscence (Burnside, 1996). While it is impossible to examine all these areas in detail, the following example, provided by a geriatric physician (Davidson, 1993, pp. 1–2), which focuses on the context of assessment and diagnosis, provides strong evidence in support of the ethical imperative to storylisten.

Several years ago, Mr. Daniel James was admitted to a surgical unit of a large urban teaching hospital for investigation and management of urinary retention. Following surgery, he became increasingly disoriented and agitated, requiring him to be both physically and chemically restrained. Shortly following this, the surgical resident in charge of his case described him as demented and likely suffering from Alzheimer's disease. He was transferred to the extended care area to await placement in a nursing home. At three o'clock in the morning, soon after his transfer, the nurse in charge called the medical resident on call to report that Mr. James was up and fully dressed, refusing to go back to bed. The resident arrived, ordered that the patient be restrained in bed and, as well, ordered a powerful tranquillizing medication to be given intramuscularly.

The following morning, the geriatric resident was called to take over responsibility of Mr. James. The resident noted that he was stuporous but appeared acutely ill. When the chart was reviewed, the resident noted that there was very little historical information, as Mr. James had arrived alone on the day of admission and was vague about his background. A sister in another city was contacted and the resident was able to begin to develop a comprehensive historical review of Mr. James's life. Of interest was the fact that Mr. James had worked all of his adult life as a milkman, and that it was his lifelong pattern to rise and dress at two forty-five in the morning. Unfortunately, it was too late for Mr. James. He died that same evening from a not uncommon side effect of the tranquillizing medication used to restrain him.

During a formal review of this patient's hospital chart, the social history documented by the original surgical resident stated only the following: "Retired, living alone, not coping according to landlady." The remainder of the intake history was quite typical of documentation seen in most areas of acute-care medicine. That is, the focus of the documentation was almost exclusively centered on the main presenting problem—in this case, urinary retention. Although this traditional system had done an exemplary job of correcting this physical problem, it had killed the patient through its inability to determine a holistic portrait of the patient.

This tragic but by no means isolated example highlights the fact that Mr. James's autonomy was not respected. That is, he was not considered as a person, but rather as an object with a set of physical symptoms (Davidson, 1991). From a biographical point of view, this outcome was avoidable, if someone had listened to his story—or more correctly, if someone had assumed that he had a story to tell, beyond his organismic, or "set of symptoms" story. This process would have revealed that Mr. James was still expressing his inside story: a specialized competency and an important source of meaning in his life, namely, being a milkman. Another ethical dimension of this situation is that Mr. James's hospital story was being coauthored by the medical staff, even though they were not aware of the implications of the story they were creating. Their personal and/or professional metaphors led to a tragedy and an example of an unethical situation.

The importance of reflecting on our own story in a biographical encounter will be addressed in the next section of this chapter.

The story of Mr. James provides an example of a context where storylistening is a prerequisite for ethically informed practice. The contribution of biography to the notions of autonomy and competence as reflected in such contexts is through the movement away from all-or-nothing definitions of these terms. Traditionally, people have been considered to be either competent or incompetent, and to either retain or relinquish their autonomy as a result of decisions made regarding this aspect of their lives. This all-or-nothing exclusive disjunction is increasingly being understood to constitute an unethical situation, due to the fact that people have a story to tell, whether it is verbal or nonverbal, or even when it needs to be told through a significant other.

The example of Mr. James is very effective in making this point. The basic insight here is that, from a biographical point of view, human behavior is never meaningless. A study by Hallberg in Sweden further illustrates the fact that people should not be considered totally incompetent or, as noted earlier, biographically inactive. Based on existentialist assumptions regarding the primacy of meaning, Hallberg's (1990) study showed that vocally disruptive behavior could be significantly reduced among severely dementing patients by, in essence, listening to their stories and by responding appropriately. (For a further powerful example, see the film *Awakenings*.)

If it is possible to listen to the stories of severely dementing persons, which amounts to respecting their continuity as persons, and thereby improve their quality of life, then we can envision many other less extreme contexts where this would also be possible and desirable. It is important to point out that it is not only the storyteller's story that can be changed for the better in these situations, but also the storylistener's personal and social story. For example, it is increasingly being acknowledged that a nursing home is able to function without chemical and physical restraint types of intervention to the benefit—in terms of dignity, autonomy, and respect—of residents, staff, and visitors alike. This constitutes a clear example of restorying, or trading our stories in and up.

GUIDELINES FOR EFFECTIVE STORYLISTENING

In Chapter 5, we introduced a range of approaches to restorying. We also discussed a set of techniques for effective storylistening. However, in addition to these strategies, three guidelines underlie an ethically informed biographical encounter. First, the basic assumptions and purpose of various approaches and programs need to be clarified and respected with regards to both training and implementation. Second, we need to make our own story available to ourselves as a prerequisite to really being able to listen to another's story. The third guideline concerns the expectations we should have when we do listen to that other story, whether it is our own or that of another person.

1. What is the purpose of the encounter?

As we saw in Chapter 5, there is a wide range of approaches to the intentional restorying of a life. A major distinction concerning these types of resources for restorying is that between therapy and learning (Alheit, 1992). Therapy-type approaches, including psychoanalysis, life-review, social work, and family therapy are designed to assist people in resolving neuroses, psychoses, and other specific conflicts. We could add support groups to this list, as they also have a focused agenda, a specific story-line or theme, whether it be alcoholism, Parkinsonism, or spousal abuse. The point here is that in all these cases the agent of restorying, usually a professional, requires a specific and appropriate type of training as an intervener. We will say more about the issue of training shortly.

However, there are many other learning-type restorying approaches that are effective and do not require the same level of, or perhaps any, formal training. These types of biographical encounters involve storytelling and storylistening but focus more on a free and mutual exchange of stories and sources of meaning in life without an underlying agenda or set theme. Earlier we called this *therapy for the sane.*

Guided autobiography is an example of this approach. While it is recommended that someone undergo this process before starting a new group, the main requirements are to be an open, caring person and to maintain an atmosphere of confidentiality and nonjudgmental acceptance—principles that must be made clear to all participants at the outset. As we mentioned in Chapter 5, the emphasis is on story*listening*. While guided autobiography and other learning approaches have clearly therapeutic outcomes in the broad sense of the term, they are not forms of therapy. The ethical implication here is that a person's quality of life can be damaged as well as enhanced through restorying, depending on the attention paid to this distinction. They presuppose, in some important ways, very different narrative environments. A nonfocused therapy is as inappropriate as a focused or misplaced analytical learning approach.

2. Whose story is it anyway?

The second guideline concerns the need to reflect carefully on our own conceptions, attitudes, or "meaning" in the biographical encounter, in order to clarify whose story is being constructed in various situations. Intervention is a process of going from what *is* to what *should be*. That is, we want someone to be better than he or she was at the outset. The difficulty and complexity, or the *dilemma of involvement,* in this process arises as a result of discovering and deciding how the new story should be written (Kenyon, 1991). Very often this process is directed by the intervener's expert story, as in the Mr. James case, where, to repeat, the storylistener becomes an expert in someone else's life. As Sankar and Gubrium (1994, p. xiv) indicate: "Attention to meaning is far more complex than simply asking open-ended questions and allowing participants to speak extemporane-ously. It requires a heightened sense of self-awareness about the researcher's personal understandings, beliefs, and world view." The same point applies in any storylistening situation. That is, there is an autobiographical dimen-sion to our activities as professionals, and as storylisteners in general, which means that we bring our basic assumptions and metaphors, or our personal as well as possibly professional stories, to a biographical encounter with a client, patient, or informant, friend or family member.

As we discussed in Chapter 5, it is not always easy to restory in this way. That is, there is resistance, for our stories have an immune system, particu-larly if they are sanctioned by professional training and specific scientific techniques. Moreover, the storylistener must not only possess a new story but *be* that new story. For example, the process of going from being an expert in another's life to being a "guide on the side" can be threatening and requires vulnerability and involvement—in other words, a willingness to be changed through storylistening.

Nevertheless, from a storied perspective, as professionals we have an ongoing ethical responsibility stemming from the fact that we are partici-pants in the research or practice situation, in which there is *my* personal story, *my* professional story, *your* story, and the story *we* are co-creating. Returning to our medical example, the social story created by Mr. James and the medical staff led to a tragic end to Mr. James's personal story. The origin of this problem was the professional and/or personal stories of the medical staff—professional stories in terms of training, and personal stories in the sense that it may have also involved ageism. Borrowing from Sankar and Gubrium (1994, p. xv), ethical problems arise "in not attending to subjects' worlds, meanings, and differences from 'their' points of view."

Conversely, biographical approaches, properly implemented, are particularly suited to meet this ethical challenge.

The central challenge here is for the storylistener to gain insight into the limits of his or her experience vis-à-vis that of the storyteller. A biographical approach increases the possibility of bridging the potential gap of "intersubjectivity" and really entering the lifeworld of the storyteller. This is particularly important in a situation where, for example, a younger person is biographically engaged with someone older. Biographical material gives a younger person access to information about aging and history; however, it is a history that has been *lived* by the older person (Ruth and Kenyon, 1996).

Biographical encounters constitute a process and involve paying attention to subtleties. For example, an ethically informed biographical approach should go beyond the collection and use of nursing home residents' lifestories to serve only the official nursing home world. Unless this occurs, "biographical particulars, such as the resident's view of life, are ultimately marginalized in organizational processing, even while enlightened administrators and staff try to take them into account" (Gubrium, 1993, p. 180). From an ethical perspective, the challenge here is to make a decision to include the resident's story in the official picture. That is, in this and other situations, the person is living and creating his or her own unique story within a particular social setting and social story. As we have discussed, creating new stories and creating a self requires a dynamic between our personal selves and other people. Problems arise when our experiences are being "storied" by others, or by ourselves, in a way that does not represent our lived experience. In the next section, we will take up some ethical issues concerning authenticity (or truth) and coherence (or completeness) in a lifestory.

A focus on subjective meaning or personal stories facilitates an environment whereby the larger intersubjective story that is coauthored in a biographical encounter will include all relevant components (all things considered), minimize isolation and separation, and enhance communion and community. If, as we are arguing here, storytelling constitutes a spiritual or existential dimension of human nature and if that dimension involves a quality of relatedness, then preventing someone from expressing his or her story and participating to the extent possible might be "among the greatest transgressions" (Boyajian, 1988, p. 21). From this point of view, storytelling might be nearly as important as eating.

However, a focus and respect for the personal dimension of stories, an approach that also respects autonomy, does not amount to the exclusion of other aspects of the biographical encounter. As Roy (1988, p. 39) notes: "As we strive to build an ethics capable of respecting personal originality, the danger to be aware of is the seduction of a facile relativism that ignores the bonds and the possibilities of our shared humanity. These bonds are the foundation for an ethics of aging." This quotation is yet another reminder that stories are created and expressed in intersubjective situations, and this in turn echoes the fact that human beings are not isolated individuals. Consequently, when we speak of autonomy and respecting personal stories, this reflects the basic ethical question presented at the outset, namely, what should I do in this situation, *all* things considered? One of the things to consider, and the most important component, is the personal story.

An example of ethically informed storylistening in practice is the work of David Roy in clinical or bedside ethics. In this approach, "the patient's biography—his or her clinical situation, relationships, life plans, beliefs, perceptions, persuasions, and total life interests—is the bottom line" (Roy, 1988, p. 32). It is evident from this example that an emphasis on a biography is not equivalent to catering only to the wishes of a particular person. In fact, as we discussed in Chapters 1 and 2, notions of autonomy and independence based on radical individualism do not reflect our storied nature, and, in fact, may represent one of our biggest problems as we enter the twenty-first century.

In practical terms, as Bould, Sanborn, and Reif (1989, p. 4) note: "Throughout most people's lives, the reality is not total independence but interdependence within the family and the community." These authors go on to say that as we age, and particularly in the case of the oldest old, our greatest need is to establish viable situations of interdependence. Interdependence permits self-determination or autonomy, while dependence results "from requiring the help of others but being unable to negotiate the terms of the help received" (p. 4). Another way to say this is that we are again concerned with negotiated consent.

3. What should we expect from storylistening?

The third guideline concerns our expectations regarding our own stories and those of others. There are four worth looking at here. The first is *universality*. This book emphasizes the desirability and even necessity of biographical approaches in various contexts. However, even though the activity of self-reflection upon self and life is a basic human capacity, an interesting ethical question is whether everyone does or ought to engage in storytelling. Is it a universal phenomenon? Should storytelling be considered a prerequisite for an authentic life, and should everyone therefore be required to engage in the process to attain mental health or some other end state?

It is interesting to note in this regard that authors such as Peter Coleman (1986) encountered people who did not have a need for reminiscence or storytelling. In working with older people, he found that some were accepting of their lives and had not, at least formally, engaged in these processes. Other current research (see Webster, 1994) suggests that in cases of such things as depression, recent trauma, and even specific personality traits, biographical forms of intervention may be experienced "as invasive, coercive, or otherwise threatening to clients who feel they have been inappropriately and/or prematurely engaged in such programs" (Webster, 1994, p. 68). There is a good practical lesson to be learned from this, namely that biographical reflections are not necessarily for everyone, nor at all times. In other words, it would not appear ethically appropriate to view storytelling and restorying as the key to successful aging or a meaningful life. There are situations when it is appropriate "not to story."

Second, there are ethical implications stemming from the idea we discussed earlier that stories are never *complete*. Neither my own story, nor the story of another, is the whole story, since that story is being looked at from a particular perspective or for a specific purpose, whether it be to collect data on how people age, to facilitate self-reflection in an intervention situation, or to understand my own life better. The important conclusion here is that it is not possible to arrive at the final truth about a life. Nevertheless, we still "know" ourselves and others and we establish our identity by learning about lifestories. As part of the quality of opacity (and contingency) built into our story, human beings do not always know the origin of events or what they can and should hold themselves responsible for.

Another reason for not being capable of complete understanding of a life story is that, as existential beings, we are unique. At some point, we are not like anyone else. Still, our stories are *genre-lizable* and, in this regard, lives can be discussed in general terms. As David Roy indicated earlier, there are ties that bind. However, even though the station-stops on our journeys may be similar, our stories are never exactly alike.

Further, as we discussed in Chapter 2, stories are not complete since it is an open question whether there is *one* story to tell. In addition to our earlier consideration of this topic, we can add Wallace (1992), who points to the same conclusion in a study in which people were asked to "just tell their story." There were no ready-made lifestories; rather, the story emerged as a function of a specific interpersonal context. Again, the courtroom demands for the truth, the whole truth, and nothing but the truth would seem misplaced when we look more closely at human interaction from a storied perspective.

As we have also discussed, the story of my life might better be termed, at least in some important ways, the *stories* I am. Individual stories or subplots need not add up to a grand narrative, either over time or at any point in time. A personally meaningful and authentic lifestory is not only created, it is also discovered. One makes an effort and hopes for a basic sense of coherence and viability. This coherence is established out of periodic confusion, incoherence, and chaos (Carr, 1986; Riegel, 1976). Moreover, to repeat a remark we made earlier, sometimes it is a case of how some event or action fits into the existing story (we lose our place in the book); other times, things are more serious as we realize that the question is now "what *is* the story?"

From an ethical perspective, these features of life as story underline the importance of compassion toward others, and of what a Buddhist, for example, would describe as being a friend to oneself. We may demand too much clarity or completeness from someone or blame ourselves for things beyond our control.

A third ethical issue crucial to storylistening is that there are clearly limitations to our freedom to choose any lifestory we desire, limitations that originate in our personal and sociocultural situations. The interesting and potentially optimistic feature of biographical aging is that we do not know in advance, or *a priori*, which parts of our story are locked in as facticity and which parts are open to possibility. As we said in the previous chapter, our lifestories, like our lives, are open-ended. Perhaps this is, in part, what we have in mind when we refer to the phrase "triumph of the human spirit." That is, one is often surprised at the story a person, including oneself, has created-discovered in dealing meaningfully with a particular life event or *way of life* (Ruth and Oberg, 1996).

Research indicates that people are able to find meaning in very severe circumstances, such as incest, cancer, or loss of a loved one; in other words, we are capable of *radical restorying*. A very powerful example of the effectiveness of storytelling is the work of Victor Frankl (1962) with survivors of the death camps. It is important to emphasize that finding meaning is more than simply uncovering some positive feature of a negative or traumatic experience. People who find meaning through restorying often report that their story and their self has changed significantly and that their lives have been enriched over the long term. Again, they not only *have* a new story, they *are* a new story. Many people who have come through events such as divorce, widowhood, serious illness, and near death experiences will say that they are actually better and happier persons than they were before the trauma. We consider further examples of radical restorying in Chapter 7.

When we consider all these existential aspects of storytelling, the business of storylistening becomes a process that truly does require listening and not just hearing another's story. As we have discussed throughout this volume, depending to some degree on the context of the biographical encounter, there is no specific version of a lifestory that would be true or genuine as opposed to false or inauthentic. Such a quest breaks the hermeneutic circle, which is a fundamental element of personal storytelling and the entire enterprise of biography. The notion of a true story implies that someone knows the truth. But we have argued that none of the characters in the story of human existence has the entire script. This situation has prompted the remark that the narrative situation is rather ironic, perhaps even a source of humor, due to the disparity of understanding between what the narrator, characters, and audience each knows about the story (Scholes and Kellogg, 1966).

As we discussed at the outset, in lifestories and narratives we are dealing with individual perceptions, attributions of meaning, and interpretations. From this perspective, a lifestory does not contain the answer to something, it *is* the answer. Thus, Carl Jung notes that what is important in his autobiography is not the truth of the stories he tells about his life in some objective sense. Rather, the only question is whether "what I tell is my fable, *my* truth" (cited in Charmé, 1984, p. 155).

Therefore, for example, whether someone lives according to a more idiosyncratic story or set of values, or a traditional story, such as a particular religious tradition, an authentic lifestory is the one that a person imbues with meaning. My meanings are not necessarily your meanings, and the storylistener should not make a priori assumptions about the contents of another's facticity or material for his or her sense of possibility, that is, his or her restorying material. Our ethical obligation to others is to respect the integrity and autonomy of another person by accepting the story that he or she chooses to live by. This is a *sine qua non* for entering the lifeworld of another.

Relating our discussion of therapy in the last chapter to an ethical context, the role of the storylistener, whether therapist, educator, spiritual counselor, concerned friend, or family member, is "not to replace one client story with another," as Gergen (1996, p. 215) points out, "but to enable clients to participate in the continuous process of creating and transforming meaning." This activity involves more than the observation of patterns or themes by the storylistener while he or she remains the expert at a distance, independent from the process. Rather, the storylistener in the biographical encounter is a collaborator and coauthor of the story. This process is captured effectively by Michael White (1991, p. 30): "The therapist can facilitate the generation and/or resurrection of alternative stories by orienting him/herself to these unique outcomes as one might orient themselves to mysteries. These are mysteries that only persons can unravel as they respond to the therapist's curiosity about them. As persons take up the task of unravelling such mysteries, they immediately engage in storytelling and meaning-making."

The fourth ethical issue concerning storylistening expectations involves the very way that we understand another's story. As we discussed in Chapter 2, properly implemented, biographical approaches can help a person to realize a basic acceptance of his or her life and thereby improve his or her *quality* of life. However, this acceptance can be perceived, observed, or assessed in a variety of ways. It might reflect a cognitively loaded notion of ego integrity, as in a written autobiography or a fully coherent life narrative. It might simply be a statement like *it was real* in reference to one's life. In other words, acceptance may not be expressed in a well thought out story. It may not even be verbal in nature but behavioral, something that can be observed in very frail people or dementing persons. The story need not be written or spoken in words. As Joseph Foley notes in discussing dementing persons, "we too often assume that the absence of emotional display means that no emotion is being experienced. We too often assume that because communication is absent, internal mental process has stopped" (cited in Callahan, 1995, p. 26).

The ethical implication here is that the demand for a good beginning, middle, and end may not reflect an accurate phenomenological description of coherence, and may place inappropriate, inordinate, and counterproductive demands on storied *human* beings. The meaning-value of personal storytelling (Kenyon, 1996a) may be at least as much a matter of intuition and feeling as it is of logic and ideas, both in terms of our own story and of our ability to understand another's. In this regard, we need to acknowledge possible limitations of the life as story metaphor, or at least acknowledge that it is possible that we may be many different types of stories.

INTERRUPTED RESTORYING OR A STALLED ITINERARY

As storied beings, or beings en route, restorying is always a possibility. However, for some people there is a closure brought to the journey or their understanding of life as a story or journey. For the disengaged or despairing person, time is closed. As Victor Frankl (1962) would say, "there is nothing to expect from life anymore." Existentialist philosopher, Gabriel Marcel (1962), would say that the person has chosen to despair, to catalogue and define life once and for all, and to disarm before the inevitable. Such a person is no longer part of his or her own lifestory. He or she has imposed an end to his or her journey. However, we would argue that it is an imposition on something that still goes on at deeper levels of the self, as well as for other people. Metaphors of rigidity, contraction, and isolation are operative here.

For storylisteners two ethical points need to be made in this context. First, periods of anxiety, confusion, and even despair are a natural part of all human lifestories. As we mentioned earlier, sometimes we may not even know what the story is. The value of these unsettling experiences is sometimes underestimated; that is, we often "fear" anxiety when it is actually a part of our growth process. During these times, it would be unethical to impose storytelling on a person or attempt to remove or prevent what is an inside part of a healing and restorying process, until there is a desire for storytelling.

Second, at the other extreme, it appears that there are people who are rather seriously hardened by life, whose closure and story is perhaps too coherent, whose facticity leaves little room for restorying or for cultivating their sense of possibility. While we do not ever know until a person dies, at least, who these candidates are—that is, there is always hope—there are severe limitations to trading in and trading up in these cases. All we can do is provide an appropriate narrative environment.

However, for most of us, biographical encounters of some form or another are beneficial, and this means that good storylisteners are of great value. We can make a big difference in each other's lives, professionally and personally, as fellow pilgrims en route, by sharing one another's journey and communicating metaphors of hope and dignity to those who are often particularly vulnerable. From a gerontologist's perspective, nowhere is this more evident than in such environments as nursing homes, where residents can be made to feel either that they are professional invalid characters in their personal and social stories, or that, as Gubrium says, they are biographically active—in other words, that they are persons with specific limitations as part of their very rich and unique lifestories.

We need to acknowledge, not that a person has become less than a full human being, but that there is a sometimes very significant change from the person who *was* there to the person who is there. In the case of a dementing person, the agent of restorying can play a crucial role by virtue of his or her own personal and social story in coauthoring the personal and social story of the vulnerable person. This is another context where it is necessary to story, even if we do not know exactly what is going on in the dementing person's mind.

CONCLUSION

Underlying all the ethical issues we have just discussed is the basic principle of listening to and accepting the story of another—moreover, a story that is "ours in the making." Given that biography is a basic element of our being in the world, the outcome of an appropriate biographical encounter is the facilitation of another person to continue on his or her journey and to find his or her own direction. Often, this result is obtained through the very process of storytelling and storylistening. Conversely, if this basic principle of biographical aging and biography is not respected, either through omission or commission, then serious ethical problems arise. It is one thing to engage in ethical dialogue in order to determine appropriate action in *this* situation, and another to ignore the ethical implications of one's actions, implications that are operative in any case. As the often quoted maxim in ethics states, to do nothing is to do something.

As a final remark, since there is a distinctively existential-spiritual dimension to the stories we are and to storylistening, all members of the encounter can be deeply changed cognitively, emotionally, and behaviorally. This sentiment is captured compellingly by Gubrium (1993, p. 187), as he reflects on a study of nursing home residents:

What was I hearing as they conveyed their experience? Data? Stories? Responses? Meanings? Interviewees? Narratives? I was hearing all of this, of course, but placed side by side, the resulting polarities shocked me. Data vs stories. Responses vs meaning. Interviewees versus storytellers. It shocked me because, on the one side, I was aiming to complete a study and, on the other, I was witnessing what the suffering and dying were telling me, were conveying for me. It was a gift, really, and it shocked me that I had to remain committed at the time to listening, recording and going about research business, respondent after respondent. It was a gift I could not return then, having to remain satisfied that only later I could give something in return by telling their stories in the best way I could.

In the next and final chapter, we will explore some implications, extensions, and speculations of our story of the life-as-story metaphor.

NOTE

1. An earlier version of this chapter appears in Kenyon, 1996b.

Chapter 7

The Journey of the Story and the Story of the Journey

The only role that's mine to play, the ultimate rule to keep, is to not forget or turn away, not to sleep through the dance.

George Fowler (1995)

INTRODUCTION

We are approaching the end of our journey into the metaphor of life as story. However, as with both a good story and a meaningful journey, there are more chapters to be written and more destinations to seek—more than we can account for here. In this chapter, then, we simply want to note a few of the many questions and speculations that this rich way of thinking suggests. First, we consider the optimistic directions for human development that the metaphor indicates; next, the relationship between stories and the proverbial wisdom of age. After that, we consider the definition of terms like wisdom and acceptance; then, the issue of older stories in the twenty-first century. Finally, we identify certain questions for further reflection and research that our journey leaves outstanding.

OPTIMISTIC DIRECTIONS FOR HUMAN DEVELOPMENT

The story metaphor raises a host of questions regarding the purpose—or teleology—of both lifestories and lives. For example, is there some kind of transition during the process of aging that brings an automatic increase in existential understanding, in wisdom or acceptance? Does the story of human development resemble a spiritually informed journey? Is there a relationship between the suffering, loss, and disillusionment that afflict the

traveler and the possibility of a movement in life from *having* to *being*?
(Kenyon, 1992). Indeed, it is just such a relationship that Florida Scott-Maxwell seems to note in this statement from her autobiography, written when
she was well into her eighties: "The hardness of life I deplore creates the
qualities I admire" (1968, p. 47).

Such questions invite philosophical speculation regarding our ontological roots. However, they invite very practical speculation as well, which has
a direct bearing on ourselves as storytellers and storylisteners, or agents of
restorying. If the idea that we *are* stories is valid, then they present a
potentially positive and hopeful direction for the human journey. That
optimism stems from the basic fact that stories are never locked in, that they
are always made up of facticity *and* possibility, and that what is possible is
not known in advance. There is an aspect of openness, therefore, even of
creativity, built into the very fabric of human life. In other words, as life
goes on, most of us *do* seem to learn a few things for the better about
ourselves, our relationships, and our world.

Two additional, related sets of issues are important to touch on in this
connection. The first concerns the links between life as story and the process
of spirituality, as understood and practiced in a number of traditions. The
second concerns the evidence that comes from several sources suggesting
that many people do indeed *live* stories of acceptance and meaning, particularly as they age. The implication is that if we look at ourselves from a
storied perspective, we will see and be capable of facilitating more positive
incidents of restorying. We will consider this second set of issues first.

An approach that provides some of the evidence in question is one we
have referred to already, namely, guided autobiography. In this minimally
directed approach to restorying, participants often become curious as to why
particular aspects of their stories do or do not become visible in the course
of sharing with group members their experience of specific themes. At one
time, that is, they highlight particular experiences in the story they relate
which, at another time, they omit. This can be rather disconcerting when
they realize that they failed to discuss a death or some other trauma, on the
one hand, or a major positive event, such as a marriage, on the other. Often,
objective events such as a war, a serious illness, a separation or exile will
not figure in a person's journey at all, at least in the way we might expect.
In other words, in telling ourselves there are always surprises.

Although in certain biographical encounters the issue of defense mecha-
nisms would be relevant, what we are seeing here may simply be an
illustration of the basic aspect of openness and creativity that characterizes
human life. Moreover, this aspect becomes more visible—this existential-

spiritual dimension reveals itself—precisely when the storytelling agenda is not set in advance, when we are simply given the opportunity to tell our story in a supportive environment without a specific focus on major life events or a particular therapeutic agenda.

The idea of openness or creativity in the story of the journey follows from our earlier discussions of the coherence, opacity, and completeness of lifestories. But it is given an additional, positive interpretation by looking at aspects of *spirituality*, broadly defined. That is, it may be quite natural for people *not* to find coherence between their present inside story and an earlier version of themselves. Elaborating this point leads us to the second set of issues.

In many spiritual traditions, such as Buddhism and Christianity, we may find through meditation and reconciliation that, as we grow, we become less and less fond of the person we have been in the past. We may find that person egotistical or narrow-minded, perhaps lacking in compassion. In Eriksonian terms, a degree of integrity may lead us to a desire for *generativity* (McAdams, 1996), meaning to a view of ourselves as a larger being with stronger desires for communion and participation than for achievement and competition. As we discussed in Chapter 5, restorying of this kind can often take place as a result of a near-death experience, of divorce or the loss of a career; from it, we emerge what to both others and ourselves seems a different person. Once again, we need only think how we feel when someone from our past insists on relating to us in terms of the story we were when we knew them before. However much we try to convince them that we are literally a different person, that we not only *have* a new story but *are* one, in our thoughts, feelings, and actions, and in the sources of meaning upon which we draw, they resist seeing and accepting the changes we have undergone.

Another interesting issue here has to do with the directionality of this restorying process: where it is leading us as storied beings, whether there are any *limits* to it, whether it is possible to restory too radically or too often. Moreover, is it an outcome meant for the lucky few, for the karmically selected, or is it a natural destination of the human journey?

These are complex questions that are not simply answered. Like all good questions, they keep coming back. In fact, as most spiritual traditions acknowledge, there is an element of mystery here, just as in stories there is always an element of opacity. All the same, it is possible to search for examples of authentic lifestories and to consider what is involved in what we commonly think of as the wisdom of age.

STORIES AND THE WISDOM OF AGE

Do people attain some degree of acceptance, meaning, or wisdom in life? If so, then how do we tell? While there is no systematic answer to such questions, the list of observations supporting the commonsense belief behind them grows longer with each day. Manheimer (1992, p. 431), for example, provides an interesting review of studies that "give dramatic form to retelling the story of late-life transformation in which disability, frailty, limitation, dependency, and despair undergo an inversion, becoming qualities such as capability, strength, possibility, autonomy, and wisdom."

Other investigations of biographical aging carried out by Kaufman (1986), Coleman (1986), and Ruth and Oberg (1996), have found that most of the older people studied attained some degree of personal meaning and life acceptance. Reker and Wong (1988) reported similar findings and added that there may be an increase in *existential understanding* in the later years of life. In a major study in 1966 focusing on attitudes toward aging, death, and dying, Dutch gerontologist Joep Munnichs reached the conclusion that older persons' attitudes reflected an *awareness of finitude*, which involved an acceptance of life coupled with a tranquility in facing death. Such a view is also echoed in the writing of Elizabeth Kubler-Ross and others who work with the terminally ill.

Other sources that have found meaning in life include the examples of radical restorying that we mentioned in Chapter 6. Important studies of this type are those carried out by Silver, Boon, and Stones (1983) and by Taylor, Wood, and Lichtman (1983) with victims of abuse, incest, and cancer. Their findings point to the ability of the human spirit, through a process of restorying, to develop, create, and discover a sense of both meaning and possibility in the midst of extreme circumstances. A further example of radical restorying is in a study by Van den Hoonaard (forthcoming) which analyzes published works written by widows and concludes that many widows *find themselves*—their own identity, their personal story—following the death of their husbands. Previously, their identity was their husband's identity; their story, his. Finally, near-death experiences are increasingly recognized as sources of radical restorying (Rinpoche, 1992).

An interesting study from a different perspective is one done by Leon Edel (1979). In an interpretation of a series of self-portraits by Rembrandt, Edel concludes that the artist painted until the very end, and that his journey terminated in an attitude of openness, acceptance, and wonder. More recently, researchers on aging have begun using a storied perspective to look at its specifically spiritual dimensions (Sherman and Webb, 1994).

In addition to these sources from formal academic research, many professionals working with older persons report similar findings. Also, in a gerontology course at St. Thomas University where undergraduates carry out a biographical interview with an older person (some four hundred have been completed to date), it is remarkable how often they report that their negative stereotypes are replaced by an attitude of respect for someone who in fact has something significant to say to them and who appears to live a meaningful lifestory.

DEFINING ACCEPTANCE AND WISDOM

But what is it that all these people are claiming to see amid such biographical encounters? We believe it to be qualities we could call acceptance and wisdom. Though we shall not attempt to offer official definitions of these phenomena here, we can describe certain characteristics of them that arise out of our previous discussion. In general, people appear to manifest wisdom and demonstrate acceptance in a wide variety of ways—once again reflecting the creative nature of storied beings.

1. Acceptance or wisdom might be expressed in an autobiography as a well-written story with a beginning, middle, and end—literally, a good novel.

2. In contrast to this highly cognitive expression of biographical aging, acceptance or integrity might be expressed in Erikson's (1979, p. 32) rendering of Dr. Borg's last stage of life, as "transcendent simplicity, rather than mystical rapture or intellectual reconstruction." Even this simplicity, however, might take a wide variety of forms. For example, a later life insight into the journey of life might be expressed as *cross-legged immobility*, as Holliday and Chandler (1986) have called it, or as intense political activity, as might be inferred about Bertrand Russell. In fact, the latter would probably be perceived as more acceptable in Western culture, where silence is anathema to most people and rest is simply unproductive time. As Moody (1991, p. 64) indicates:

So we can easily feel a sentimental pity toward the old when they are unable or unwilling to share those reflexes of haste and superficiality that have become our daily habits. In our common desire to help the elderly, what we secretly wish is to prolong the haste that excludes us from even a moment of quietness and contemplation. We find the quietness of the old, even their very presence, disturbing, as if it were a repudiation of all that we hold dear.

3. Less obvious expressions of the stories we are are captured in statements such as "survival with grace." As Mary Frances Fisher notes, "We like old people who have aged well, because of what we experience as their reassuring warmth of amusement" (cited in Weisbord, 1990, p. 156).

4. As we said earlier, in the case of a frail or dementing person, acceptance might amount simply to a look of serenity or acceptance. Despite the difficulty in categorizing instances of acceptance and wisdom in later life, a common feature of this phenomenon is that a person is able to view his or her life *as* a story; in other words, there is a degree of self-transcendence, a space between his or her story and his or her "self." In journey terms, he or she is able to watch the scenery of life as from the window of a train. This means that a person has seen through certain things about himself or herself, has "read" his or her own story and those of other people. There is an attitude of detachment evident here; however, it is combined with an active concern with life. In studying spirituality in older person's stories, Sherman and Webb (1994, pp. 259–260) found that most people, "most certainly did display a 'letting-go' quality and an acceptance of their inevitable losses, but they definitely cannot be described as 'resigned.' They appeared to be in a state of being that was quite alive, but that was also more contemplative than they described themselves as being in earlier life stages." Further, this acceptance often involves a sense of humor about ourselves and the world. Following Erikson, "I can't imagine a wise old person who can't laugh. The world is full of ridiculous dichotomies" (cited in Weisbord, 1990, p.156).

A general conclusion we can draw, then, from our exploration of the stories we are, is that we know very little about the limits of the human spirit. To repeat one of our basic themes, we must be careful not to assume that a particular person, including oneself, is locked in by his or her facticity or is permanently stalled in his or her journey, that he or she cannot restory or is too old to change. As Aftel (1996, p. 174) notes, "some plots seem to be so powerful that they create themselves over and over, and you fear you will never be able to change them." Yet, the examples above and many others besides would indicate that we do not know what, if any, stories lock a person in permanently. There appears to be always room for hope, for cultivating our sense of possibility, and for confirming our ability to restory, even though the process must begin with our own personal, inside story. As Aftel puts it:

Sometimes it is our unexamined assumptions about life that do us in: the idea that long-term relationships inevitably become stale or humdrum; that living with a teenager is hell; that life goes downhill after forty. It is very important to look at seldom-examined ideas like these. To creatively rewrite our narratives, we need all the freedom to redescribe our lives that we can get. Weeding out assumptions of this kind gives us more freedom to use poetic license when writing our plots. (1996, p. 175)

OLDER STORIES IN THE TWENTY-FIRST CENTURY

With reference to Moody's remark concerning age and quietness, do we need to learn silence and rest from older stories? Are the stories of older persons a possible partial remedy to the negative outcomes of postmodern society that we discussed in earlier chapters? This may be, insofar as older stories point to sources of meaning and purpose in life and move us away from viewing aging in exclusively technical terms—that is, as a problem to be solved. The key question here, both individually and culturally, is whether science is capable of even asking, let alone answering, questions that pertain to the human quest for love and meaning in the face of death.

Throughout this volume, we have attempted to address the main problem faced by postmodern persons and cultures, namely that of separateness or of a lack of relatedness in its various forms. An interesting question here is whether older stories, with their lessons of acceptance and *ordinary wisdom* (see Randall and Kenyon, in preparation), could be of great value if we were disposed to storylisten as the first step in our restorying process. In other words, do we have a need to engage in a process of *reclaiming* the wisdom of age?

OUTSTANDING QUESTIONS

We draw this book to a close with a clustering of further questions that hang with us as we approach the frontier to which our journey has led.

If emotions have narrative roots, then how does our emotional life change as we undergo radical restorying? In questioning the ways we have storied our lives in the past, do we open ourselves to a whole different set of emotions—or to none at all perhaps, to a state of flatness or emotionlessness amid the relative *de*-storying, or storylessness, that the reading phase involves? What generally are the connections between our emotional life and our autobiographical development?

If there is such a thing as narrative intelligence, then do some of us have more of it than others? If so, what are the implications of such differences for how we story our lives, and the extent to which we can be open to restorying? Furthermore, what are the links between the level of our narrative intelligence and our ability to "read" our lives—that is, to learn autobiographically—and between our narrative intelligence and wisdom, understood as the message or meaning that any good story mediates?

If, as we believe, the story metaphor provides a comparatively safe space in which different fields within the broad realm of the human sciences can discourse concerning the *inside*—and the interconnectedness—of human development, then how is such a discourse to proceed? By whose rules? To what end? And how will we fare through the battle of (discipline-d) stories that we are unlikely to avoid along the way?

If other people are forever coauthoring us (as we are them), then what are the dynamics and the dangers of the conflict stirred up inside us as different people story us in different directions—parents this way, spouses that way, friends another way, therapists another way still?

If self-reading is essential to restorying, then what about generations to come, who may be so computer-dependent that they are "illiterate" in terms of the *deep* reading required and stimulated by a literary novel? (See Birkerts, 1994.) Might ours be the last generation interested in personal growth at all, in autobiographical reflection, in telling our stories and listening to those of others?

If intentionally telling ourselves (to others or ourselves, on paper or in conversation) is central to restorying, then how are we changed by getting our story out? How does the process of turning ourselves inside-out this thoroughly (transforming experience into expression) change our very relationship to our "self," as to others around us? How might the increased sensitivity to the nuances and details, the flicks and darts of our inner world, affect our involvement in the changes of our outer one—make us too detached or too obsessive, too introspective, too anal, or too self-aware?

If we story our lives within a web of larger stories still, or if the texts of our lives are endlessly entwined with those of others and other systems, then who are "we"? This question concerns not only the construction of personal identity (Gergen, 1991) but also the issue of personal responsibility, both ethical and legal. Moreover, given the problematic relationship between lifestory and life, it concerns how we distinguish sanity from insanity, normal from abnormal, and how we define and determine conditions like delusion, self-deception, or dissociation.

If a lifestory thickens as it unfolds, then does it not at some point narrow as well—like any novel, becoming feebler the nearer it reaches its end (Forster, 1962)? If so, then what are the implications of such a perspective for how we view conditions we might refer to as senility or second childhood? (See Prado, 1986.) Is there a possibility that we can be further along on a lifestory line and yet feel younger, as in narratively more vulnerable, just as readers become more involved in a story and more held by its allure, the more of it they read? Furthermore, what are the implications of this perspective for how we assess what is a good lifestory or a good old age? Finally, might it not lead us to a new appreciation for the novelty of each life from beginning to end, taking the course of human evolution in an essentially uncharted direction?

If each of us has a distinctive storying style, then can we still also be "genre-lizable" in ways stories are considered to be? If so, in what are such genres rooted: in the larger stories by which we have been authored, in the type of narrative intelligence we possess, or in the genes with which we were born? And how deeply can we expect ourselves to re-genre-ate in the course of restorying, or is it a case of "once a tragedian always a tragedian"?

Lastly, is re-genre-ation necessarily good? For instance, is a *tragic* lifestory automatically bad? Does each genre not have its own integrity? Should a genre-al variety not be encouraged, in support of the proverbial spice of life? If all *literary* stories were comedies or adventures, for example, would something not be lost? In a totalitarian (or authoritarian) society, is this perhaps not the *real* tragedy, that only a limited range of life-scripts are allowed, with all others seen as *sub*-versions of the dominant myth?

CONCLUSION

These questions are all jumping-off places, pointing to the next round of reflections on the life-as-story metaphor. However, we return here to the implicit question with which we embarked on this book: Can we be our own best therapists? Our answer is, much of the time, yes. Accordingly, we have sketched a perspective we call "therapoetics," or therapy for the sane. Therapy for the sane involves problem-solving and a return to a basic equilibrium of some kind, yes; but it also celebrates the possibility for wholeness, for being more than we think we are, for having peak experiences, for recovering lost dreams, and for playing the rewarding role of coauthoring in the lives of each other.

In this respect, the metaphor of life as story—specifically of *restorying*—is implicitly empowering. It can certainly inspire us as we seek meaning and strength in the face of the large scale structural changes that impact our lives in today's world and by which we are invariably, though variously, shaped—depending on our personal facticity and sense of possibility. For this reason, perhaps the appropriate phrase to invoke as we embark on intentionally restorying our lives is that we be granted the serenity to accept what we cannot change, the courage to change what we can, and the wisdom to know the difference.

References

Aftel, M. (1996). *The Story of Your Life: Becoming the Author of Your Experience*. New York: Simon and Schuster.

Alheit, P. (1992). "The Biographical Approach to Adult Education." In W. Mader (ed.), *Adult Education in the Federal Republic of Germany: Scholarly Approaches and Professional Practice*. Vancouver: The University of British Columbia Press.

———. (1995). "Biographical Learning: Theoretical Outline, Challenges and Contradictions of a New Approach in Adult Education." In P. Alheit, A. Bron-Wojciechowska, E. Brugger, and P. Dominice (eds.), *The Biographical Approach in European Adult Education*. Vienna: Verband Wiener Volksbildung. 57–74.

Allen, W. (1949). *Writers on Writing*. London: E. P. Dutton.

Atkinson, R. (1995). *The Gift of Stories: Practical and Spiritual Applications of Autobiography, Life Stories, and Personal Mythmaking*. Westport, CT: Bergin and Garvey.

Barthes, R. ([1968] 1990). "The Death of the Author." In D. Walder (ed.), *Literature in the Modern World: Critical Essays and Documents*. Oxford: Oxford University Press. 228–232.

Bateson, M. (1989). *Composing a Life*. New York: Atlantic Monthly Press.

———. (1993). "Composing a Life." In C. Simpkinson and A. Simpkinson (eds.), *Sacred Stories: A Celebration of the Power of Stories to Transform and Heal*. San Francisco: HarperCollins. 39–52.

Beach, R. (1990). "The Creative Development of Meaning: Using Autobiographical Experiences to Interpret Literature." In D. Bogdan and S. Straw (eds.), *Beyond Communication: Reading Comprehension and Criticism*. Portsmouth, NH: Boynton/Cook Heinemann. 211–235.

Belenky, M., B. Clinchy, N. Goldberger, and J. Tarule (1986). *Women's Ways of Knowing: The Development of Self, Voice, and Mind*. New York: Basic Books.

Berger, P. (1963). *Invitation to Sociology: A Humanistic Perspective*. Garden City, NJ: Anchor Books.

Bianchi, E. (1995). *Aging as a Spiritual Journey*. New York: Crossroad.

Birkerts, S. (1994). *The Gutenberg Elegies: The Fate of Reading in an Electronic Age*. New York: Fawcett.

Birren, J. (1987). "The Best of All Stories," *Psychology Today* (May). 74–75.

Birren, J., and B. Birren (1996). "Autobiography: Exploring the Self and Encouraging Development." In J. Birren, G. Kenyon, J.-E. Ruth, J. Schroots, and T. Svensson (eds.), *Aging and Biography: Explorations in Adult Development*. New York: Springer. 283–299.

Birren, J., and D. Deutchman (1991). *Guiding Autobiography Groups for Older Adults: Exploring the Fabric of Life*. Baltimore: Johns Hopkins University Press.

Birren, J., G. Kenyon, J-E. Ruth, J. Schroots, and T. Svensson (eds.) (1996). *Aging and Biography: Explorations in Adult Development*. New York: Springer.

Birren, J. and W. Schaie (eds.) (1996). *Handbook of the Psychology of Aging*. 4th ed. San Diego: Academic Press.

Blythe, R. (1979). *The View in Winter: Reflections on Old Age*. London: Penguin.

Boetzkes, E. (1993). "Autonomy and Advance Directives." *Canadian Journal on Aging*, 12 (4). 441–452.

Booth, W. (1966). "Types of Narration." In R. Scholes (ed.), *Approaches to the Novel*. San Francisco: Chandler. 273–290.

———. (1988). *The Company We Keep: An Ethics of Fiction*. Berkeley: University of California Press.

Botella, L., and G. Feixas (1993). "The Autobiographical Group: A Tool for the Reconstruction of Past Life Experiences with the Aged." *International Journal of Aging and Human Development*, 36 (4). 303–319.

Bould, S., B. Sanborn, and L. Reif (1989). *Eighty-five Plus: The Oldest Old*. Belmont, CA: Wadsworth.

Boyajian, J. (1988). "On Reaching a New Agenda: Self-Determination and Aging." In J. Thornton and E. Winkler (eds.), *Ethics and Aging*. Vancouver: University of British Columbia Press. 16–30.

Brady, E. (1990). "Redeemed from Time: Learning Through Autobiography." *Adult Education Quarterly* 41 (1). 43–52.

Bridges, W. (1980). *Transitions: Making Sense of Life's Changes*. Toronto: Addison-Wesley.

Brooks, P. (1985). *Reading for the Plot: Design and Intention in Narrative*. New York: Vintage.

Bruner, E. (1986). "Experience and Its Expressions." In V. Turner and E. Bruner (eds.), *The Anthropology of Experience*. Urbana, IL: University of Illinois Press. 3–30.

Bruner, J. (1983). *In Search of Mind: Essays in Autobiography.* New York: Harper and Row.

————. (1986). *Actual Minds, Possible Worlds.* Cambridge, MA: Harvard University Press.

————. (1987). "Life as Narrative." *Social Research,* 54 (1). 11–32.

————. (1990). *Acts of Meaning.* Cambridge, MA: Harvard University Press.

Bruner, J., and S. Weisser (1991). "The Invention of Self: Autobiography and Its Forms." In D. Olson and N. Torrance (eds.), *Literacy and Orality.* Cambridge: Cambridge University Press. 129–148.

Burnside, I. (1996). "Life Review and Reminiscence in Nursing Practice." In J. Birren, G. Kenyon, J-E. Ruth, J. Schroots, and T. Svensson (eds.). *Aging and Biography: Explorations in Adult Development.* New York: Springer. 248–264.

Butler, R. (1963). "The Life-Review: An Interpretation of Reminiscence in the Aged." *Psychiatry,* 26. 63–76.

Callahan, D. (1995). "Terminating Life-Sustaining Treatment of the Demented." *Hastings Center Report,* 25 (6). 25–31.

Campbell, J., and B. Moyers (1988). *The Power of Myth.* New York: Doubleday.

Carr, D. (1986). *Time, Narrative, and History.* Bloomington, Indiana University Press.

Casey, E. (1987). *Remembering: A Phenomenological Study.* Bloomington: Indiana University Press.

Castaneda, C. (1975). *Journey to Ixtlan: The Lessons of Don Juan.* London: Penguin.

Charmé, S. (1984). *Meaning and Myth in the Study of Lives: A Sartrean Perspective.* Philadelphia: University of Pennsylvania Press.

Chatman, S. (1978). *Story and Discourse.* Ithaca, NY: Cornell University Press.

Checkland, D., and M. Silberfeld. (1993). "Competence and the Three A's: Autonomy, Authenticity, and Aging." *Canadian Journal on Aging,* 12(4). 453–468.

Cohler, B., and T. Cole (1996). "Studying Older Lives: Reciprocal Acts of Telling and Listening." In J. Birren, G. Kenyon, J-E. Ruth, J. Schroots, and T. Svensson (eds.), *Aging and Biography: Explorations in Adult Development.* New York: Springer. 61–76.

Cole, T. (1992). *The Journey of Life.* New York: Cambridge University Press.

Cole, T., D. van Tassel, and R. Kastenbaum (eds.) (1992). *Handbook of the Humanities and Aging.* New York: Springer.

Coleman, P. (1986). *Ageing and Reminiscence Processes.* New York: Wiley.

Coles, R. (1989). *The Call of Stories: Teaching and the Moral Imagination.* Boston: Houghton Mifflin.

Connelly, E., and D. Clandinin (1988). *Teachers as Curriculum Planners: Narratives of Experience.* New York: Teachers College Press.

Crisp, J. (1995). "Making Sense of the Stories that People with Alzheimer's Tell: A Journey with My Mother." *Nursing Inquiry*, 2. 133–140.

Crites, S. (1971). "The Narrative Quality of Experience." *Journal of the American Academy of Religion*, 39 (3). 291–311.

Csikszentimihalyi, M., and O. Beattie (1979). "Life Themes: A Theoretical and Empirical Exploration of Their Origins and Effects. "*Journal of Humanistic Psychology*, 19(1). 45–63.

Cupitt, D. (1991). *What Is a Story?* London: SCM Press.

Daloz, L. (1986). *Effective Teaching and Mentoring: Realizing the Transformational Power of Adult Learning Experiences.* San Francisco: Jossey-Bass.

Danto, A. (1985). *Narration and Knowledge.* New York: Columbia University Press.

Davidson, W. (1991). "Metaphors of Health and Aging: Geriatrics as Metaphor." In G. Kenyon, J. Birren, and J. Schroots (eds.), *Metaphors of Aging in Science and the Humanities.* New York: Springer. 173–184.

————. (1993). "Utility and Implications of Comprehensive Personal Biography in Clinical Geriatric Medicine." Paper presented at the annual meeting of the Gerontological Society of America, New Orleans, Louisiana.

de Beauvoir, S. (1973). *The Coming of Age.* New York: Warner.

Eakin, P. (1985). *Fictions in Autobiography: Studies in the Art of Self-Invention,* Princeton: Princeton University Press.

Edel, L. (1979). "Portrait of the Artist as an Old Man." In D. van Tassel (ed.), *Aging, Death, and the Completion of Being.* Philadelphia: University of Pennsylvania Press. 193–214.

Elias, J., and S. Merriam (1980). *Philosophical Foundations of Adult Education.* Malabar, FL: Krieger.

Engel, M. (1972). Preface. In G. Bateson, *Steps to an Ecology of Mind.* New York: Ballantine. vii–viii.

Erikson, E. (1963). *Childhood and Society.* New York: Norton.

————. (1979). "Reflections on Dr. Borg's Life Cycle." In D. van Tassel (ed.), *Aging, Death, and the Completion of Being.* Philadelphia: University of Pennsylvania Press. 29–67.

Feinstein, D., S. Krippner, and D. Granger (1988). "Mythmaking and Human Development." *Journal of Humanistic Psychology*, 28(3). 23–50.

Field, J. (1952). *A Life of One's Own.* London: Penguin.

Fischer, L. (1994). "Qualitative Research as Art and Science." In J. Gubrium and A. Sankar (eds.), *Qualitative Methods in Aging Research.* Thousand Oaks, CA: Sage. 3–14.

Flynn, D. (1991). "Community as Story: A Comparative Study of Community in Canada, England, and the Netherlands." *The Rural Sociologist*, Spring. 24–35.

Forster, E. (1962). *Aspects of the Novel.* London: Penguin.

Fowler, G. (1995). *Dance of a Fallen Monk*. New York: Addison-Wesley.

Fowler, J. (1981). *Stages of Faith: The Psychology of Human Development and the Quest for Meaning*. San Francisco: Harper and Row.

Frankl, V. (1962). *Man's Search for Meaning*. New York: Simon and Schuster.

Frye, J. (1986). *Living Stories, Telling Lives: Women and the Novel in Contemporary Experience*. Ann Arbor, University of Michigan Press.

Frye, N. (1963). *The Educated Imagination*. Toronto: CBC.

————. (1966). "Fictional Modes and Forms." In R. Scholes (ed.), *Approaches to the Novel*. San Francisco: Chandler. 23–42.

————. (1988). *On Education*. Toronto: Fitzhenry and Whiteside.

Gadamer, H. (1976). *Philosophical Hermeneutics*. Berkeley, CA: University of California Press.

Gardner, H. (1990). *Frames of Mind: The Theory of Multiple Intelligences*. San Francisco: Basic Books.

Gardner, J. (1978). *On Moral Fiction*. New York: Basic Books.

————. (1985). *The Art of Fiction: Notes on Craft for Young Writers*. New York: Vintage.

Gearing, B., and P. Coleman (1996). "Biographical Assessment in Community Care." In J. Birren, G. Kenyon, J.-E. Ruth, J. Schroots, and T. Svensson (eds.), *Aging and Biography: Explorations in Adult Development*. New York: Springer. 265–282.

Gergen, K. (1986). "Narrative Form and the Construction of Psychological Science." In T. Sarbin (ed.), *Narrative Psychology: The Storied Nature of Human Conduct*. New York: Praeger. 22–44.

————. (1991). *The Saturated Self*. New York: Basic Books.

————. (1996). "Beyond Life Narratives in the Therapeutic Encounter." In J. Birren, G. Kenyon, J-E. Ruth, J. Schroots, and T. Svensson (eds.), *Aging and Biography: Explorations in Adult Development*. New York: Springer. 205–223.

Gergen, K., and M. Gergen (1983). "Narratives of the Self." In T. Sarbin and E. Schiebe (eds.), *Studies in Social Identity*. New York: Praeger. 254–273.

Gergen, K., and M. Gergen (1986). "Narrative Form and the Construction of Psychological Science." In T. Sarbin (ed.), *Narrative Psychology: The Storied Nature of Human Conduct*. New York: Praeger. 22–43.

Gergen, M., and K. Gergen (1984). "The Social Construction of Narrative Accounts." In K. Gergen and M. Gergen (eds.), *Historical Social Psychology*. Hillsdale, NJ: Lawrence Erlbaum. 173–189.

Gilligan, C. (1982). *In a Different Voice*. Cambridge, MA: Harvard University Press.

Glover, J. (1988). *I: The Philosophy and Psychology of Personal Identity*. London: Penguin.

Goffman, E. (1959). *The Presentation of Self in Everyday Life*. New York: Doubleday Anchor.

Gold, J. (1990). *Read for Your Life: Literature as a Life Support System.* Markham, ON: Fitzhenry and Whiteside.

Greene, M. (1990). "The Emancipatory Power of Literature." In J. Mezirow (ed.), *Fostering Critical Reflection in Adulthood.* San Francisco: Jossey-Bass. 251–268.

Gubrium, J. (1993). *Speaking of Life: Horizons of Meaning for Nursing Home Residents.* Hawthorne, NY: Aldine de Gruyter.

————. (1995). "Individual Agency, the Ordinary and Postmodern Life." Inaugural Lecture, Centre for Ageing and Biographical Studies, School of Health and Social Welfare, The Open University, England.

Haight, B., and J. Webster (eds.) (1995). *The Art and Science of Reminiscing: Theory, Research, Methods, and Applications.* Washington, DC: Taylor and Francis.

Hall, E. (1984). *The Dance of Life: The Other Dimension of Time.* New York: Doubleday.

Hallberg, L. (1990). "Vocally Disruptive Behaviour in Severely Demented Patients in Relation to Institutional Care Provided." *Umea University Medical Dissertations*, Umea, Sweden.

Harrison, C. (1993). "Personhood, Dementia and the Integrity of a Life." *Canadian Journal on Aging*, 12 (4). 428–440.

Hauerwas, S. (1977). *Truthfulness and Tragedy: Further Investigations into Christian Ethics.* Notre Dame, IN: University of Notre Dame Press.

Hauerwas, S., and L. Jones (eds.) (1989). *Why Narrative? Readings in Narrative Theology.* Grand Rapids, MI: Eerdmans.

Havelock, E. (1991). "The Oral-Literate Equation: A Formula for the Modern Mind." In D. Olson and N. Torrance (eds.), *Literacy and Orality.* New York: Cambridge University Press. 11–27.

Heilbrun, C. (1988). *Writing a Woman's Life.* New York: Ballantine.

Hillman, J. (1975). "The Fiction of Case History: A Round." In J. Wiggins (ed.), *Religion as Story.* New York: Harper and Row. 123–173.

————. (1989). *A Blue Fire.* New York: Harper and Row.

Hodgins, J. (1993). *A Passion for Narrative: A Guide for Writing Fiction.* Toronto: McClelland and Stewart.

Holliday, S., and M. Chandler (1986). *Wisdom: Explorations in Adult Competence.* Basel: Karger.

Hopkins, R. (1994). *Narrative Schooling: Experiential Learning and the Transformation of American Education.* New York: Teachers College Press.

Horner, J. (1982). *That Time of Year: A Chronicle of Life in a Nursing Home.* Amherst: University of Massachusetts Press.

Houston, J. (1987). *The Search for the Beloved: Journeys in Sacred Psychology.* Los Angeles: Jeremy P. Tarcher.

Kaufman, S. (1986). *The Ageless Self: Sources of Meaning in Late Life.* New York: New American Library.

Kayser-Jones, J., and B. Koenig (1994). "Ethical Issues." In J. Gubrium and A. Sankar (eds.), *Qualitative Methods in Aging Research.* Thousand Oaks, CA: Sage.

Kazin, A. (1981). "The Self as History: Reflections on Autobiography." In A. Stone (ed.), *The American Autobiography: A Collection of Critical Essays.* Englewood Cliffs, NJ: Prentice-Hall. 31–43.

Keen, E. (1986). "Paranoia and Cataclysmic Narratives." In T. Sarbin (ed.), *Narrative Psychology: The Storied Nature of Human Conduct.* New York: Praeger. 174–190.

Keen, S. (1988). "The Stories We Live By." *Psychology Today* (December). 42–47.

———. (1993). "On Mythic Stories." In C. Simpkinson and A. Simpkinson (eds.), *Sacred Stories: A Celebration of the Power of Stories to Transform and Heal.* San Francisco: HarperCollins. 27–37.

Keen, S., and A. Fox (1974). *Telling Your Story: A Guide to Who You Are and Who You Can Be.* Toronto: New American Library.

Kegan, R. (1982). *The Evolving Self.* Cambridge, MA: Harvard University Press.

Kennedy, E. (1976). *The Joy of Being Human.* New York: Image.

Kenyon, G. (1980). "The Meaning of Death in Gabriel Marcel's Philosophy." *Gnosis* 2(1). 27–40.

———. (1988). "Basic Assumptions in Theories of Human Aging." In J. Birren and V. Bengtson (eds.), *Emergent Theories of Aging.* New York: Springer. 3–18.

———. (1991). "*Homo Viator*: Metaphors of Aging, Authenticity, and Meaning." In G. Kenyon, J. Birren, and J. Schroots (eds.), *Metaphors of Aging in Science and the Humanities.* New York: Springer. 17–35.

———. (1992). "Aging and Possibilities for Being." *Aging and the Human Spirit*, 2(1). 4–5.

———. (1996a). "The Meaning Value of Personal Storytelling." In J. Birren, G. Kenyon, J.-E. Ruth, J. Schroots, and T. Svensson (eds.), *Aging and Biography: Explorations in Adult Development.* New York: Springer. 21–38.

———. (1996b). "Ethical Issues in Ageing and Biography." *Ageing and Society.* 16(6).

Kenyon, G., J. Birren, and J. Schroots (eds.) (1991). *Metaphors of Aging in Science and the Humanities.* New York: Springer.

Kenyon, G., and W. Davidson (1993). "Ethics in an Aging Society." In *Ethics and Aging. Writings in Gerontology*, No. 13. Ottawa: National Advisory Council on Aging.

Kerby, A. (1991). *Narrative and the Self.* Bloomington: Indiana University Press.

Kermode, F. (1966). *The Sense of an Ending: Studies in the Theory of Fiction.* New York: Oxford University Press.

————. (1980). "Secrets and Narrative Sequence." In W. Mitchell (ed.), *On Narrative*. Chicago: University of Chicago Press. 79–97.

Kotre, J. (1990). *Outliving the Self: Generativity and the Interpretation of Lives*. Baltimore: Johns Hopkins University Press.

Laing, R. (1967). *The Politics of Experience*. New York: Ballantine.

Lakoff, G., and M. Johnson (1980). *Metaphors We Live By*. Chicago: University of Chicago Press.

Larsen, S. (1990). *The Mythic Imagination: Your Quest for Meaning Through Personal Mythology*. New York: Bantam.

Leakey, R., and R. Lewin (1978). *People of the Lake: Mankind and Its Beginnings*. New York: Avon.

Le Guin, U. (1989). *Dancing at the Edge of the World: Thoughts on Words, Women, Places*. New York: Harper and Row.

Leitch, T. (1986). *What Stories Are: Narrative Theory and Interpretation*. University Park: Pennsylvania State University Press.

Lejeune, P. (1989). *On Autobiography*. Minneapolis: University of Minnesota Press.

Leonard, J. (1994). "Not Losing Her Memory: Stories in Photographs, Words and Collage." *Modern Fiction Studies*, 40 (3). 657–685.

Lewis, C. (1966). "On Stories." In *Essays Presented to Charles Williams*. Grand Rapids, MI: Eerdmans. 90–105.

Linde, C. (1993). *Life Stories: The Creation of Coherence*. New York: Oxford University Press.

Loori, J. (1993). "The Zen Koan: Lancet of Self-Inquiry." In C. Simpkinson and A. Simpkinson (eds.), *Sacred Stories: A Celebration of the Power of Stories to Transform and Heal*. San Francisco: HarperCollins. 191–207.

Lubbock, P. ([1921] 1965). *The Craft of Fiction*. London: Jonathan Cape.

Maddi, S. (1988). "On the Problem of Accepting Facticity and Pursuing Possibility." In S. Messer, L. Sass, and R. Woolfolk (eds.), *Hermeneutics and Psychological Theory*. New Brunswick, NJ: Rutgers University Press. 182–209.

Mader, W. (1991). "Aging and the Metaphor of Narcissism." In G. Kenyon, J. Birren, and J. Schroots (eds.), *Metaphors of Aging in Science and the Humanities*. New York: Springer. 131–153.

Mader, W. (1995). "Thematically Guided Autobiographical Reconstruction: On Theory and Method of 'Guided Autobiography' in Adult Education." In P. Alheit, A. Bron-Wojciechowska, E. Brugger, and Dominicé (eds.), *The Biographical Approach in Adult Education*. Vienna: Verband Wiener Volksbildung. 244–257.

————. (1996). "Emotionality and Continuity in Biographical Contexts." In J. Birren, G. Kenyon, J-E. Ruth, J. Schroots, and T. Svensson (eds.), *Aging and Biography: Explorations in Adult Development*. New York: Springer. 39–60.

Mancusco, J., and T. Sarbin (1983). "The Self-Narrative in the Enactment of Roles." In T. Sarbin and E. Schiebe (eds.), *Studies in Social Identity*. New York: Praeger. 233–253.

Manheimer, R. (1992). "Wisdom and Method: Philosophical Contributions to Gerontology." In T. Cole, D. van Tassel, and R. Kastenbaum (eds.), *Handbook of the Humanities and Aging*. New York: Springer. 426–440.

Marcel, G. (1962). *Homo Viator*. New York: Harper and Row.

Maugham, W. S. (1938). *The Summing Up*. New York: Mentor.

McAdams, D. (1988). *Power, Intimacy, and the Life-Story: Personological Inquiries into Identity*. New York: Guilford.

———. (1994). *The Person: An Introduction to Personality Psychology*, 2d ed. New York: Harcourt Brace.

———. (1996). "Narrating the Self in Adulthood." In J. Birren, G. Kenyon, J.-E.Ruth, J. Schroots, and T. Svensson (eds.), *Aging and Biography: Explorations in Adult Development*. New York: Springer. 131–148.

Mezirow, J. (1978). "Perspective Transformation." *Adult Education*, 28(2). 100–110.

Monette, P. (1992). *Becoming a Man: Half a Life Story*. San Francisco: Harper San Francisco.

Moody, H. (1988). "From Informed Consent to Negotiated Consent" (Special Supplement on Autonomy and Long-Term Care). *Gerontologist*, 28. 64–70.

———. (1991). "The Meaning of Life in Old Age." In N. Jecker (ed.), *Aging and Ethics*. Clifton, NJ: Humana. 51–92.

Moore, T. (1992). *Care of the Soul: A Guide for Cultivating Depth and Sacredness in Everyday Life*. New York: HarperCollins.

Moustakas, C. (1967). *Creativity and Conformity*. New York: Van Nostrand Reinhold.

Munnichs, J. (1966). *Old Age and Finitude*. Basel: Karger.

Murray, K. (1989). "The Construction of Identity in the Narratives of Romance and Comedy." In J. Shotter and K. Gergen (eds.), *Texts of Identity*. London: Sage. 176–205.

Napier, N. (1993). "Living Our Stories: Discovering and Replacing Limiting Family Myths." In C. Simpkinson and A. Simpkinson (eds.), *Sacred Stories: A Celebration of the Power of Stories to Transform and Heal*. San Francisco: Harper San Francisco. 143–156.

Neisser, U. (1986). "Nested Structure in Autobiographical Memory." In D. Rubin (ed.), *Autobiographical Memory*. New York: Cambridge University Press. 71–81.

Niebuhr, H. (1941). *The Meaning of Revelation*. New York: Macmillan.

Novak, M. (1971). *Ascent of the Mountain, Flight of the Dove*. New York: Harper and Row.

Nussbaum, M. (1989). "Narrative Emotions: Beckett's Genealogy of Love." In S. Hauerwas and L. Jones (eds.), *Why Narrative?: Readings in Narrative Theology*. Grand Rapids, MI: Eerdmans. 216–248.

Ochberg, R. (1995). "Life Stories and Storied Lives." In A. Lieblich and R. Josselson (eds.), *Exploring Identity and Gender: The Narrative Study of Lives, vol. 2*. London: Sage. 113–144.

Olney, J. (ed.). (1980). *Autobiography: Essays Theoretical and Critical*. Princeton: Princeton University Press.

Ortony, A. (ed.) (1979). *Metaphor and Thought*. Cambridge: Cambridge University Press.

Owen, H. (1987). *Spirit: Transformation and the Development of Organizations*. Potomac, MD: Abbott.

Parry, A., and R. Doan (1994). *Story Re-visions: Narrative Therapy in the Postmodern World*. New York: Guilford Press.

Pascal, R. (1960). *Design and Truth in Autobiography*. London: Routledge and Kegan Paul.

Pearson, C. (1989). *The Hero Within: Six Archetypes We Live By*. San Francisco: Harper and Row.

Pennebaker, J. (1990). *Opening Up: The Healing Power of Confiding in Others*. New York: Avon.

Plank, W. (1989). *Gulag 65: A Humanist Looks at Aging*. New York: Peter Lang.

Polkinghorne, D. (1988). *Narrative Knowing and the Human Sciences*. Albany: SUNY Press.

————. (1996). "Narrative Knowing and the Study of Lives." In J. Birren, G. Kenyon, J-E. Ruth, J. Schroots, and T. Svensson (eds.), *Aging and Biography: Explorations in Adult Development*. New York: Springer. 77–99

Polonoff, D. (1987). "Self-deception." *Social Research*, 54(1). 45–53.

Polster, E. (1987). *Every Person's Life Is Worth a Novel*. New York: Norton.

Prado, C. (1986). *Rethinking How We Age*. Westport, CT: Greenwood.

Prince, G. (1987). *A Dictionary of Narratology*. Lincoln: University of Nebraska Press.

Progoff, I. (1975). *At a Journal Workshop: The Basic Guide and Text for Using the Intensive Journal*. New York: Dialogue House Library.

Rainer, T. (1978). *The New Diary*. Los Angeles: Jeremy P. Tarcher.

Randall, W. (1995). *The Stories We Are: An Essay on Self-Creation*. Toronto: University of Toronto Press.

————. (1996). "Restorying a Life: Adult Education and Transformative Learning." In J. Birren, G. Kenyon, J.-E. Ruth, J. Schroots, and T. Svensson (eds.), *Aging and Biography: Explorations in Adult Development*. New York: Springer. 224–247.

Randall, W., and G. Kenyon (in preparation). *Ordinary Wisdom: Biographical Aging and the Journey of Life*.

Reker, G., and P. Wong (1988). "Aging as an Individual Process: Toward a Theory of Personal Meaning." In J. Birren and V. Bengtson (eds.), *Emergent Theories of Aging.* New York: Springer. 214–246.

Ricoeur, P. (1980). "Narrative Time." In W. Mitchell (ed.), *On Narrative.* Chicago: University of Chicago Press. 165–186.

Riegel, K. (1976). "The Dialectics of Human Development." *American Psychologist,* 31. 689–700.

Rinpoche, S. (1992). *The Tibetan Book of Living and Dying.* London: Random House.

Rosen, H. (1986). "The Importance of Story." *Language Arts,* 63(3). 226–237.

Rosenau, P. (1992). *Post-Modernism and the Social Sciences: Insights, Inroads, and Intrusions.* Princeton: Princeton University Press.

Roy, D. (1988). "Ethics and Aging: Trends and Problems in the Clinical Setting." In J. Thornton and E. Winkler (eds.), *Ethics and Aging.* Vancouver: University of British Columbia Press. 31–40.

Rubin, D. (ed.) (1986). *Autobiographical Memory.* New York: Cambridge University Press.

Runyan, W. (1984). *Life Histories and Psychobiography: Explorations in Theory and Method.* New York: Oxford University Press.

Ruth, J.-E., and G. Kenyon (1996). "Biography in Adult Development and Aging." In J. Birren, G. Kenyon, J.-E. Ruth, J. Schroots, and T. Svensson (eds.), *Aging and Biography: Explorations in Adult Development.* New York: Springer. 1–20.

Ruth, J.-E., and P. Oberg (1996). "Ways of Life: Old Age in a Life History Perspective." In J. Birren, G. Kenyon, J.-E. Ruth, J. Schroots, and T. Svensson (eds.), *Aging and Biography: Explorations in Adult Development.* New York: Springer. 167–186.

Ruth, J.-E., and A. Vilkko (1996). "Emotions in the Construction of Autobiography." In C. Magai and S. H. McFadden (eds.), *Handbook of Emotion, Adult Development, and Aging.* New York: Academic Press. 167–181.

Sacks, O. (1985). *The Man Who Mistook His Wife for a Hat, and Other Clinical Tales.* New York: Summit.

Salaman, E. (1982). "A Collection of Moments." In U. Neisser. (ed.), *Memory Observed: Remembering in Natural Contexts.* San Francisco: W. H. Freeman. 49–63.

Sankar, A., and J. Gubrium (1994). Introduction. In J. Gubrium and A. Sankar (eds.), *Qualitative Methods in Aging Research.* Thousand Oaks, CA: Sage.

Sarbin, T. (ed.) (1986a). *Narrative Psychology: The Storied Nature of Human Conduct.* New York: Praeger.

———. (1986b). "The Narrative as a Root Metaphor for Psychology." In T. Sarbin (ed.), *Narrative Psychology: The Storied Nature of Human Conduct.* New York: Praeger. 3–21.

182 References

Sartre, J. (1955). *No Exit and Three Other Plays*. New York: Knopf.

———. (1956). *Being and Nothingness*. New York: Simon and Schuster.

———. ([1938] 1965). *Nausea*. London: Penguin.

Schacter, D. (1996). *Searching for Memory: The Brain, the Mind, and the Past*. New York: Basic Books.

Schafer, R. (1980). "Narration in the Psychoanalytic Dialogue." In W. Mitchell (ed.), *On Narrative*. Chicago: University of Chicago Press. 25–49.

———. (1983). *The Analytic Attitude*. New York: Basic Books.

———. (1989). "The Sense of an Answer: Ambiguities of Interpretation in Clinical and Applied Psychoanalysis." In R. Cohen (ed.), *The Future of Literary Theory*. New York: Routledge. 188–207.

———. (1992). *Retelling a Life: Narrative and Dialogue in Psychoanalysis*. New York: Basic Books.

Schank, R. (1990). *Tell Me a Story: A New Look at Real and Artificial Memory*. New York: Scribner's.

Schnitzer, P. (1993). "Tales of the Absent Father: Applying the 'Story' Metaphor in Family Therapy." *Family Process*, 32. 441–458.

Scholes, R., and R. Kellogg (1966). *The Nature of Narrative*. New York: Oxford University Press.

Schroots, J., J. Birren, and G. Kenyon (1991). "Metaphors and Aging: An Overview." In G. Kenyon, J. Birren, and J. Schroots (eds.), *Metaphors of Aging in Science and the Humanities*. New York: Springer. 1–16.

Scott-Maxwell, F. (1968). *The Measure of My Days*. London: Penguin.

Sherman, E., and T. Webb (1994). "The Self as Process in Late-Life Reminiscence: Spiritual Attributes." *Ageing and Society*, 14. 255–267.

Shotter, J., and K. Gergen (eds.) (1989). *Texts of Identity*. London: Sage.

Silver, R., C. Boon, and M. Stones (1983). "Searching for Meaning in Misfortune: Making Sense of Incest." *Journal of Social Issues*, 39(2). 81–102.

Singer, P. (1979). *Practical Ethics*. New York: Cambridge University Press.

Skinner, B. (1983). *A Matter of Consequences: Part Three of an Autobiography*. New York: Knopf.

Smith, S. (1987). *A Poetics of Women's Autobiography: Marginality and the Fictions of Self-Representation*. Bloomington: Indiana University Press.

Spence, D. (1982). *Narrative Truth and Historical Truth*. New York: W. W. Norton.

Steele, R. (1986). "Deconstructing History: Toward a Systematic Criticism of Psychological Narratives." In T. Sarbin (ed.), *Narrative Psychology: The Storied Nature of Human Conduct*. Westport, CT: Praeger. 256–275.

Stone, A. (ed.) (1981). *The American Autobiography: A Collection of Critical Essays*. Englewood Cliffs, NJ: Prentice-Hall.

Stone, E. (1988). *Black Sheep and Kissing Cousins: How Our Family Stories Shape Us*. London: Penguin.

Stroup, G. (1981). *The Promise of Narrative Theology*. Atlanta: John Knox.

Tannen, D. (1990). *You Just Don't Understand: Women and Men in Conversation.* New York: Ballantine.

Taylor, S., J. Wood, and R. Lichtman (1983). "It Could Be Worse: Selective Evaluation as a Response to Victimization." *Journal of Social Issues,* 39(2). 19–40.

TeSelle, S. (1975). *Speaking in Parables: A Study in Metaphor and Theology.* Philadelphia: Fortress.

Tilley, T. (1985). *Story Theology.* Wilmington, DE: Michael Glazier.

Truitt, A. (1987). *Turn: The Journal of an Artist.* London: Penguin.

Turner, V., and E. Bruner (eds.) (1986). *The Anthropology of Experience.* Chicago: University of Illinois Press.

Van den Hoonaard, D. (forthcoming). "Identity Foreclosure: Women's Experiences of Widowhood in Autobiographical Accounts." *Ageing and Society.*

Van den Hoonaard, D. (in preparation). *A Different Life: Older Women's Experiences of Widowhood.* Waterloo, ON: Wilfred Laurier University Press.

Vargiu, J. (1978). "Subpersonalities." *Synthesis,* 1. 60–63, 73–89.

Wallace, B. (1992). "Reconsidering the Life Review: The Social Construction of Talk About the Past." *Gerontologist,* 32(1). 120–125.

Webster, J. (1994). "Predictors of Reminiscence: A Lifespan Perspective." *Canadian Journal on Aging.* 13(1). 66–78.

Weisbord, M. (1990). *Our Future Selves.* Toronto: Random House.

White, H. (1980). "The Value of Narrativity in the Representation of Reality." In W. Mitchell (ed.), *On Narrative.* Chicago: University of Chicago Press. 1–23.

White, M. (1991). "Deconstruction and Therapy." *Dulwich Centre Newsletter,* 3. 2–40.

————. (1995). *Re-authoring Lives: Interviews and Essays.* Adelaide, AU: Dulwich Centre Publications.

White, M., and D. Epston (1990). *Narrative Means to Therapeutic Ends.* New York: Norton.

Wiggins, J. (ed.) (1975). *Religion as Story.* New York: Harper and Row.

Winquist, T. (1980). *Practical Hermeneutics: A Revised Agenda for the Ministry.* Chico, CA: Scholars Press.

Witherell, C., and N. Noddings (eds.) (1991). *Stories Lives Tell: Narrative and Dialogue in Education.* New York: Teachers College Press.

Wolfe, T. (1983). *The Autobiography of an American Novelist.* Cambridge, MA: Harvard University Press.

Wyatt, F. (1986). "The Narrative in Psychoanalysis: Psychoanalytic Notes on Storytelling, Listening, and Interpreting." In. T. Sarbin (ed.), *Narrative Psychology: The Storied Nature of Human Conduct.* New York: Praeger. 193–210.

Zemke, R. (1990). "Storytelling: Back to a Basic." *Training.* 44–50.

Zweig, P. (1974). *The Adventurer.* New York: Basic Books.

Index

About the Authors

GARY M. KENYON is Director of Gerontology, St. Thomas University.

WILLIAM L. RANDALL is Research Associate to the Chair in Gerontology, St. Thomas University.

Both professors have taught and published extensively in the area of personal development.

ISBN 0-275-95663-6

HARDCOVER BAR CODE